THE OFFICIAL PARENT'S SOURCEBOOK *on*

MEGALENCEPHALY

JAMES N. PARKER, M.D.
AND PHILIP M. PARKER, PH.D., EDITORS

ICON Health Publications
ICON Group International, Inc.
4370 La Jolla Village Drive, 4th Floor
San Diego, CA 92122 USA

Printed in the United States of America.

Last digit indicates print number: 10 9 8 7 6 4 5 3 2 1

Publisher, Health Care: Philip Parker, Ph.D.
Editor(s): James Parker, M.D., Philip Parker, Ph.D.

Publisher's note: The ideas, procedures, and suggestions contained in this book are not intended as a substitute for consultation with your child's physician. All matters regarding your child's health require medical supervision. As new medical or scientific information becomes available from academic and clinical research, recommended treatments and drug therapies may undergo changes. The authors, editors, and publisher have attempted to make the information in this book up to date and accurate in accord with accepted standards at the time of publication. The authors, editors, and publisher are not responsible for errors or omissions or for consequences from application of the book, and make no warranty, expressed or implied, in regard to the contents of this book. Any practice described in this book should be applied by the reader in accordance with professional standards of care used in regard to the unique circumstances that may apply in each situation, in close consultation with a qualified physician. The reader is advised to always check product information (package inserts) for changes and new information regarding dose and contraindications before administering any drug or pharmacological product. Caution is especially urged when using new or infrequently ordered drugs, herbal remedies, vitamins and supplements, alternative therapies, complementary therapies and medicines, and integrative medical treatments.

Cataloging-in-Publication Data

Parker, James N., 1961-
Parker, Philip M., 1960-

The Official Parent's Sourcebook on Megalencephaly: A Revised and Updated Directory for the Internet Age/James N. Parker and Philip M. Parker, editors

p. cm.

Includes bibliographical references, glossary and index.

ISBN: 0-597-84114-4

1. Megalencephaly-Popular works. I. Title.

Disclaimer

Copyright Notice

Dedication

To the healthcare professionals dedicating their time and efforts to the study of megalencephaly.

Acknowledgements

The collective knowledge generated from academic and applied research summarized in various references has been critical in the creation of this sourcebook which is best viewed as a comprehensive compilation and collection of information prepared by various official agencies which directly or indirectly are dedicated to megalencephaly. All of the *Official Parent's Sourcebooks* draw from various agencies and institutions associated with the United States Department of Health and Human Services, and in particular, the Office of the Secretary of Health and Human Services (OS), the Administration for Children and Families (ACF), the Administration on Aging (AOA), the Agency for Healthcare Research and Quality (AHRQ), the Agency for Toxic Substances and Disease Registry (ATSDR), the Centers for Disease Control and Prevention (CDC), the Food and Drug Administration (FDA), the Healthcare Financing Administration (HCFA), the Health Resources and Services Administration (HRSA), the Indian Health Service (IHS), the institutions of the National Institutes of Health (NIH), the Program Support Center (PSC), and the Substance Abuse and Mental Health Services Administration (SAMHSA). In addition to these sources, information gathered from the National Library of Medicine, the United States Patent Office, the European Union, and their related organizations has been invaluable in the creation of this sourcebook. Some of the work represented was financially supported by the Research and Development Committee at INSEAD. This support is gratefully acknowledged. Finally, special thanks are owed to Tiffany Freeman for her excellent editorial support.

About the Editors

James N. Parker, M.D.

Dr. James N. Parker received his Bachelor of Science degree in Psychobiology from the University of California, Riverside and his M.D. from the University of California, San Diego. In addition to authoring numerous research publications, he has lectured at various academic institutions. Dr. Parker is the medical editor for the *Official Parent's Sourcebook* series published by ICON Health Publications.

Philip M. Parker, Ph.D.

Philip M. Parker is the Eli Lilly Chair Professor of Innovation, Business and Society at INSEAD (Fontainebleau, France and Singapore). Dr. Parker has also been Professor at the University of California, San Diego and has taught courses at Harvard University, the Hong Kong University of Science and Technology, the Massachusetts Institute of Technology, Stanford University, and UCLA. Dr. Parker is the associate editor for the *Official Parent's Sourcebook* series published by ICON Health Publications.

About ICON Health Publications

In addition to megalencephaly, *Official Parent's Sourcebooks* are available for the following related topics:

- The Official Patient's Sourcebook on Anencephaly
- The Official Patient's Sourcebook on Holoprosencephaly
- The Official Patient's Sourcebook on Hydranencephaly
- The Official Patient's Sourcebook on Hydrocephalus
- The Official Patient's Sourcebook on Lissencephaly
- The Official Patient's Sourcebook on Microcephaly
- The Official Patient's Sourcebook on Porencephaly
- The Official Patient's Sourcebook on Schizencephaly

To discover more about ICON Health Publications, simply check with your preferred online booksellers, including Barnes&Noble.com and Amazon.com which currently carry all of our titles. Or, feel free to contact us directly for bulk purchases or institutional discounts:

ICON Group International, Inc.
4370 La Jolla Village Drive, Fourth Floor
San Diego, CA 92122 USA
Fax: 858-546-4341
Web site: **www.icongrouponline.com/health**

Table of Contents

INTRODUCTION

Overview

Dr. C. Everett Koop, former U.S. Surgeon General, once said, "The best prescription is knowledge."[1] The Agency for Healthcare Research and Quality (AHRQ) of the National Institutes of Health (NIH) echoes this view and recommends that all parents incorporate education into the treatment process. According to the AHRQ:

> Finding out more about your [child's] condition is a good place to start. By contacting groups that support your [child's] condition, visiting your local library, and searching on the Internet, you can find good information to help guide your decisions for your [child's] treatment. Some information may be hard to find—especially if you don't know where to look.[2]

As the AHRQ mentions, finding the right information is not an obvious task. Though many physicians and public officials had thought that the emergence of the Internet would do much to assist parents in obtaining reliable information, in March 2001 the National Institutes of Health issued the following warning:

> The number of Web sites offering health-related resources grows every day. Many sites provide valuable information, while others may have information that is unreliable or misleading.[3]

---

[1] Quotation from **http://www.drkoop.com**.
[2] The Agency for Healthcare Research and Quality (AHRQ): **http://www.ahcpr.gov/consumer/diaginfo.htm**.
[3] From the NIH, National Cancer Institute (NCI): **http://cancertrials.nci.nih.gov/beyond/evaluating.html**.

Since the late 1990s, physicians have seen a general increase in parent Internet usage rates. Parents frequently enter their children's doctor's offices with printed Web pages of home remedies in the guise of latest medical research. This scenario is so common that doctors often spend more time dispelling misleading information than guiding children through sound therapies. *The Official Parent's Sourcebook on Megalencephaly* has been created for parents who have decided to make education and research an integral part of the treatment process. The pages that follow will tell you where and how to look for information covering virtually all topics related to megalencephaly, from the essentials to the most advanced areas of research.

The title of this book includes the word "official." This reflects the fact that the sourcebook draws from public, academic, government, and peer-reviewed research. Selected readings from various agencies are reproduced to give you some of the latest official information available to date on megalencephaly.

Given parents' increasing sophistication in using the Internet, abundant references to reliable Internet-based resources are provided throughout this sourcebook. Where possible, guidance is provided on how to obtain free-of-charge, primary research results as well as more detailed information via the Internet. E-book and electronic versions of this sourcebook are fully interactive with each of the Internet sites mentioned (clicking on a hyperlink automatically opens your browser to the site indicated). Hard copy users of this sourcebook can type cited Web addresses directly into their browsers to obtain access to the corresponding sites. Since we are working with ICON Health Publications, hard copy *Sourcebooks* are frequently updated and printed on demand to ensure that the information provided is current.

In addition to extensive references accessible via the Internet, every chapter presents a "Vocabulary Builder." Many health guides offer glossaries of technical or uncommon terms in an appendix. In editing this sourcebook, we have decided to place a smaller glossary within each chapter that covers terms used in that chapter. Given the technical nature of some chapters, you may need to revisit many sections. Building one's vocabulary of medical terms in such a gradual manner has been shown to improve the learning process.

We must emphasize that no sourcebook on megalencephaly should affirm that a specific diagnostic procedure or treatment discussed in a research study, patent, or doctoral dissertation is "correct" or your child's best option. This sourcebook is no exception. Each child is unique. Deciding on appropriate options is always up to parents in consultation with their children's physicians and healthcare providers.

Organization

This sourcebook is organized into three parts. Part I explores basic techniques to researching megalencephaly (e.g. finding guidelines on diagnosis, treatments, and prognosis), followed by a number of topics, including information on how to get in touch with organizations, associations, or other parent networks dedicated to megalencephaly. It also gives you sources of information that can help you find a doctor in your local area specializing in treating megalencephaly. Collectively, the material presented in Part I is a complete primer on basic research topics for megalencephaly.

Part II moves on to advanced research dedicated to megalencephaly. Part II is intended for those willing to invest many hours of hard work and study. It is here that we direct you to the latest scientific and applied research on megalencephaly. When possible, contact names, links via the Internet, and summaries are provided. It is in Part II where the vocabulary process becomes important as authors publishing advanced research frequently use highly specialized language. In general, every attempt is made to recommend "free-to-use" options.

Part III provides appendices of useful background reading covering megalencephaly or related disorders. The appendices are dedicated to more pragmatic issues facing parents. Accessing materials via medical libraries may be the only option for some parents, so a guide is provided for finding local medical libraries which are open to the public. Part III, therefore, focuses on advice that goes beyond the biological and scientific issues facing children with megalencephaly and their families.

Scope

While this sourcebook covers megalencephaly, doctors, research publications, and specialists may refer to your child's condition using a variety of terms. Therefore, you should understand that megalencephaly is often considered a synonym or a condition closely related to the following:

- 742.4 Other Specified Anomalies of Brain

In addition to synonyms and related conditions, physicians may refer to megalencephaly using certain coding systems. The International Classification of Diseases, 9th Revision, Clinical Modification (ICD-9-CM) is the most commonly used system of classification for the world's illnesses. Your physician may use this coding system as an administrative or tracking tool. The following classification is commonly used for megalencephaly:[4]

- macrencephaly

For the purposes of this sourcebook, we have attempted to be as inclusive as possible, looking for official information for all of the synonyms relevant to megalencephaly. You may find it useful to refer to synonyms when accessing databases or interacting with healthcare professionals and medical librarians.

Moving Forward

Since the 1980s, the world has seen a proliferation of healthcare guides covering most illnesses. Some are written by parents, patients, or their family members. These generally take a layperson's approach to understanding and coping with an illness or disorder. They can be uplifting, encouraging, and highly supportive. Other guides are authored by physicians or other healthcare providers who have a more clinical outlook. Each of these two styles of guide has its purpose and can be quite useful.

As editors, we have chosen a third route. We have chosen to expose you to as many sources of official and peer-reviewed information as practical, for the purpose of educating you about basic and advanced knowledge as recognized by medical science today. You can think of this sourcebook as your personal Internet age reference librarian.

Why "Internet age"? When their child has been diagnosed with megalencephaly, parents will often log on to the Internet, type words into a search engine, and receive several Web site listings which are mostly irrelevant or redundant. Parents are left to wonder where the relevant information is, and how to obtain it. Since only the smallest fraction of information dealing with megalencephaly is even indexed in search engines, a non-systematic approach often leads to frustration and disappointment.

[4] This list is based on the official version of the World Health Organization's 9th Revision, International Classification of Diseases (ICD-9). According to the National Technical Information Service, "ICD-9CM extensions, interpretations, modifications, addenda, or errata other than those approved by the U.S. Public Health Service and the Health Care Financing Administration are not to be considered official and should not be utilized. Continuous maintenance of the ICD-9-CM is the responsibility of the federal government."

With this sourcebook, we hope to direct you to the information you need that you would not likely find using popular Web directories. Beyond Web listings, in many cases we will reproduce brief summaries or abstracts of available reference materials. These abstracts often contain distilled information on topics of discussion.

While we focus on the more scientific aspects of megalencephaly, there is, of course, the emotional side to consider. Later in the sourcebook, we provide a chapter dedicated to helping you find parent groups and associations that can provide additional support beyond research produced by medical science. We hope that the choices we have made give you and your child the most options in moving forward. In this way, we wish you the best in your efforts to incorporate this educational approach into your child's treatment plan.

The Editors

PART I: THE ESSENTIALS

ABOUT PART I

Part I has been edited to give you access to what we feel are "the essentials" on megalencephaly. The essentials typically include a definition or description of the condition, a discussion of who it affects, the signs or symptoms, tests or diagnostic procedures, and treatments for disease. Your child's doctor or healthcare provider may have already explained the essentials of megalencephaly to you or even given you a pamphlet or brochure describing the condition. Now you are searching for more in-depth information. As editors, we have decided, nevertheless, to include a discussion on where to find essential information that can complement what the doctor has already told you. In this section we recommend a process, not a particular Web site or reference book. The process ensures that, as you search the Web, you gain background information in such a way as to maximize your understanding.

CHAPTER 1. THE ESSENTIALS ON MEGALENCEPHALY: GUIDELINES

Overview

Official agencies, as well as federally funded institutions supported by national grants, frequently publish a variety of guidelines on megalencephaly. These are typically called "Fact Sheets" or "Guidelines." They can take the form of a brochure, information kit, pamphlet, or flyer. Often they are only a few pages in length. The great advantage of guidelines over other sources is that they are often written with the parent in mind. Since new guidelines on megalencephaly can appear at any moment and be published by a number of sources, the best approach to finding guidelines is to systematically scan the Internet-based services that post them.

The National Institutes of Health (NIH)[5]

The National Institutes of Health (NIH) is the first place to search for relatively current guidelines and fact sheets on megalencephaly. Originally founded in 1887, the NIH is one of the world's foremost medical research centers and the federal focal point for medical research in the United States. At any given time, the NIH supports some 35,000 research grants at universities, medical schools, and other research and training institutions, both nationally and internationally. The rosters of those who have conducted research or who have received NIH support over the years include the world's most illustrious scientists and physicians. Among them are 97 scientists who have won the Nobel Prize for achievement in medicine.

---

[5] Adapted from the NIH: **http://www.nih.gov/about/NIHoverview.html**.

There is no guarantee that any one Institute will have a guideline on a specific medical condition, though the National Institutes of Health collectively publish over 600 guidelines for both common and rare disorders. The best way to access NIH guidelines is via the Internet. Although the NIH is organized into many different Institutes and Offices, the following is a list of key Web sites where you are most likely to find NIH clinical guidelines and publications dealing with megalencephaly and associated conditions:

- Office of the Director (OD); guidelines consolidated across agencies available at **http://www.nih.gov/health/consumer/conkey.htm**
- National Library of Medicine (NLM); extensive encyclopedia (A.D.A.M., Inc.) with guidelines available at **http://www.nlm.nih.gov/medlineplus/healthtopics.html**
- National Institute of Neurological Disorders and Stroke (NINDS); **http://www.ninds.nih.gov/health_and_medical/disorder_index.htm**

Among the above, the National Institute of Neurological Disorders and Stroke (NINDS) is particularly noteworthy. The mission of the NINDS is to reduce the burden of neurological disease—a burden borne by every age group, by every segment of society, by people all over the world.[6] To support this mission, the NINDS conducts, fosters, coordinates, and guides research on the causes, prevention, diagnosis, and treatment of neurological disorders and stroke, and supports basic research in related scientific areas. The following patient guideline was recently published by the NINDS on megalencephaly.

What Are Cephalic Disorders?[7]

Cephalic disorders are congenital conditions that stem from damage to, or abnormal development of, the budding nervous system. Cephalic is a term that means "head" or "head end of the body." Congenital means the disorder is present at, and usually before, birth. Although there are many congenital developmental disorders, this fact sheet briefly describes only cephalic conditions.

---

[6] This paragraph has been adapted from the NINDS: **http://www.ninds.nih.gov/about_ninds/mission.htm**. "Adapted" signifies that a passage has been reproduced exactly or slightly edited for this book.

[7] Adapted from the National Institute of Neurological Disorders and Stroke (NINDS): **http://www.ninds.nih.gov/health_and_medical/pubs/cephalic_disorders.htm**.

Cephalic disorders are not necessarily caused by a single factor, but may be influenced by hereditary or genetic conditions, or by environmental exposures during pregnancy such as medication taken by the mother, maternal infection, or exposure to radiation. Some cephalic disorders occur when the cranial sutures (the fibrous joints that connect the bones of the skull) join prematurely. Most cephalic disorders are caused by a disturbance that occurs very early in the development of the fetal nervous system.

The human nervous system develops from a small, specialized plate of cells on the surface of the embryo. Early in development, this plate of cells forms the neural tube, a narrow sheath that closes between the third and fourth weeks of pregnancy to form the brain and spinal cord of the embryo. Four main processes are responsible for the development of the nervous system: cell proliferation, the process in which nerve cells divide to form new generations of cells; cell migration, the process in which nerve cells move from their place of origin to the place where they will remain for life; cell differentiation, the process during which cells acquire individual characteristics; and cell death, a natural process in which cells die. Understanding the normal development of the human nervous system, one of the research priorities of the National Institute of Neurological Disorders and Stroke, may lead to a better understanding of cephalic disorders.

Damage to the developing nervous system is a major cause of chronic, disabling disorders and, sometimes, death in infants, children, and even adults. The degree to which damage to the developing nervous system harms the mind and body varies enormously. Many disabilities are mild enough to allow those afflicted to eventually function independently in society. Others are not. Some infants, children, and adults die, others remain totally disabled, and an even larger population is partially disabled, functioning well below normal capacity throughout life.

What Are the Different Types of Cephalic Disorders?

Anencephaly

Anencephaly is a neural tube defect that occurs when the cephalic (head) end of the neural tube fails to close, usually between the 23rd and 26th days of pregnancy, resulting in the absence of a major portion of the brain, skull, and scalp. Infants with this disorder are born without a forebrain - the largest part of the brain consisting mainly of the cerebrum, which is responsible for thinking and coordination. The remaining brain tissue is often exposed - not covered by bone or skin.

Infants born with anencephaly are usually blind, deaf, unconscious, and unable to feel pain. Although some individuals with anencephaly may be born with a rudimentary brainstem, the lack of a functioning cerebrum permanently rules out the possibility of ever gaining consciousness. Reflex actions such as respiration (breathing) and responses to sound or touch may occur. The disorder is one of the most common disorders of the fetal central nervous system. Approximately 1,000 to 2,000 American babies are born with anencephaly each year. The disorder affects females more often than males.

The cause of anencephaly is unknown. Although it is believed that the mother's diet and vitamin intake may play a role, scientists agree that many other factors are also involved.

There is no cure or standard treatment for anencephaly and the prognosis for affected individuals is poor. Most infants do not survive infancy. If the infant is not stillborn, then he or she will usually die within a few hours or days after birth. Anencephaly can often be diagnosed before birth through an ultrasound examination.

Recent studies have shown that the addition of folic acid to the diet of women of childbearing age may significantly reduce the incidence of neural tube defects. Therefore it is recommended that all women of childbearing age consume 0.4 mg of folic acid daily.

Colpocephaly

Colpocephaly is a disorder in which there is an abnormal enlargement of the occipital horns - the posterior or rear portion of the lateral ventricles (cavities or chambers) of the brain. This enlargement occurs when there is an underdevelopment or lack of thickening of the white matter in the posterior cerebrum. Colpocephaly is characterized by microcephaly (abnormally small head) and mental retardation. Other features may include motor abnormalities, muscle spasms, and seizures.

Although the cause is unknown, researchers believe that the disorder results from an intrauterine disturbance that occurs between the second and sixth months of pregnancy. Colpocephaly may be diagnosed late in pregnancy, although it is often misdiagnosed as hydrocephalus (excessive accumulation of cerebrospinal fluid in the brain). It may be more accurately diagnosed after birth when signs of mental retardation, microcephaly, and seizures are present.

There is no definitive treatment for colpocephaly. Anticonvulsant medications can be given to prevent seizures, and doctors try to prevent contractures (shrinkage or shortening of muscles). The prognosis for individuals with colpocephaly depends on the severity of the associated conditions and the degree of abnormal brain development. Some children benefit from special education.

Holoprosencephaly

Holoprosencephaly is a disorder characterized by the failure of the prosencephalon (the forebrain of the embryo) to develop. During normal development the forebrain is formed and the face begins to develop in the fifth and sixth weeks of pregnancy. Holoprosencephaly is caused by a failure of the embryo's forebrain to divide to form bilateral cerebral hemispheres (the left and right halves of the brain), causing defects in the development of the face and in brain structure and function.

There are three classifications of holoprosencephaly. Alobar holoprosencephaly, the most serious form in which the brain fails to separate, is usually associated with severe facial anomalies. Semilobar holoprosencephaly, in which the brain's hemispheres have a slight tendency to separate, is an intermediate form of the disease. Lobar holoprosencephaly, in which there is considerable evidence of separate brain hemispheres, is the least severe form. In some cases of lobar holoprosencephaly, the patient's brain may be nearly normal.

Holoprosencephaly, once called arhinencephaly, consists of a spectrum of defects or malformations of the brain and face. At the most severe end of this spectrum are cases involving serious malformations of the brain, malformations so severe that they are incompatible with life and often cause spontaneous intrauterine death. At the other end of the spectrum are individuals with facial defects - which may affect the eyes, nose, and upper lip - and normal or near-normal brain development. Seizures and mental retardation may occur.

The most severe of the facial defects (or anomalies) is cyclopia, an abnormality characterized by the development of a single eye, located in the area normally occupied by the root of the nose, and a missing nose or a nose in the form of a proboscis (a tubular appendage) located above the eye.

Ethmocephaly is the least common facial anomaly. It consists of a proboscis separating narrow-set eyes with an absent nose and microphthalmia (abnormal smallness of one or both eyes). Cebocephaly, another facial anomaly, is characterized by a small, flattened nose with a single nostril situated below incomplete or underdeveloped closely set eyes.

The least severe in the spectrum of facial anomalies is the median cleft lip, also called premaxillary agenesis.

Although the causes of most cases of holoprosencephaly remain unknown, researchers know that approximately one-half of all cases have a chromosomal cause. Such chromosomal anomalies as Patau's syndrome (trisomy 13) and Edwards' syndrome (trisomy 18) have been found in association with holoprosencephaly. There is an increased risk for the disorder in infants of diabetic mothers.

There is no treatment for holoprosencephaly and the prognosis for individuals with the disorder is poor. Most of those who survive show no significant developmental gains. For children who survive, treatment is symptomatic. It is possible that improved management of diabetic pregnancies may help prevent holoprosencephaly, however there is no means of primary prevention.

Hydranencephaly

Hydranencephaly is a rare condition in which the cerebral hemispheres are absent and replaced by sacs filled with cerebrospinal fluid. Usually the cerebellum and brainstem are formed normally. An infant with hydranencephaly may appear normal at birth. The infant's head size and spontaneous reflexes such as sucking, swallowing, crying, and moving the arms and legs may all seem normal. However, after a few weeks the infant usually becomes irritable and has increased muscle tone (hypertonia). After several months of life, seizures and hydrocephalus may develop. Other symptoms may include visual impairment, lack of growth, deafness, blindness, spastic quadriparesis (paralysis), and intellectual deficits.

Hydranencephaly is an extreme form of porencephaly (a rare disorder, discussed later in this fact sheet, characterized by a cyst or cavity in the cerebral hemispheres) and may be caused by vascular insult or injuries, infections, or traumatic disorders after the 12th week of pregnancy.

Diagnosis may be delayed for several months because the infant's early behavior appears to be relatively normal. Transillumination, an examination in which light is passed through body tissues, usually confirms the diagnosis. Some infants may have additional abnormalities at birth including seizures, myoclonus (involuntary sudden, rapid jerks), and respiratory problems.

There is no standard treatment for hydranencephaly. Treatment is symptomatic and supportive. Hydrocephalus may be treated with a shunt.

The outlook for children with hydranencephaly is poor. Death generally occurs before age 1.

Iniencephaly

Iniencephaly is a rare neural tube defect that combines extreme retroflexion (backward bending) of the head with severe defects of the spine. The affected infant tends to be short, with a disproportionately large head. Diagnosis can be made immediately after birth because the head is so severely retroflexed that the face looks upward. The skin of the face is connected directly to the skin of the chest and the scalp is directly connected to the skin of the back. Generally, the neck is absent.

Most individuals with iniencephaly have other associated anomalies such as anencephaly, cephalocele (a disorder in which part of the cranial contents protrudes from the skull), hydrocephalus, cyclopia, absence of the mandible (lower jaw bone), cleft lip and palate, cardiovascular disorders, diaphragmatic hernia, and gastrointestinal malformation. The disorder is more common among females.

The prognosis for those with iniencephaly is extremely poor. Newborns with iniencephaly seldom live more than a few hours. The distortion of the fetal body may also pose a danger to the mother's life.

Lissencephaly

Lissencephaly, which literally means "smooth brain," is a rare brain formation disorder characterized by microcephaly and the lack of normal convolutions (folds) in the brain. It is caused by defective neuronal migration, the process in which nerve cells move from their place of origin to their permanent location.

The surface of a normal brain is formed by a complex series of folds and grooves. The folds are called gyri or convolutions, and the grooves are called sulci. In children with lissencephaly, the normal convolutions are absent or only partly formed, making the surface of the brain smooth.

Symptoms of the disorder may include unusual facial appearance, difficulty swallowing, failure to thrive, and severe psychomotor retardation. Anomalies of the hands, fingers, or toes, muscle spasms, and seizures may also occur.

Lissencephaly may be diagnosed at or soon after birth. Diagnosis may be confirmed by ultrasound, computed tomography (CT), or magnetic resonance imaging (MRI).

Lissencephaly may be caused by intrauterine viral infections or viral infections in the fetus during the first trimester, insufficient blood supply to the baby's brain early in pregnancy, or a genetic disorder. There are two distinct genetic causes of lissencephaly - X-linked and chromosome 17-linked.

The spectrum of lissencephaly is only now becoming more defined as neuroimaging and genetics has provided more insights into migration disorders. Other causes which have not yet been identified are likely as well.

Lissencephaly may be associated with other diseases including isolated lissencephaly sequence, Miller-Dieker syndrome, and Walker-Warburg syndrome.

Treatment for those with lissencephaly is symptomatic and depends on the severity and locations of the brain malformations. Supportive care may be needed to help with comfort and nursing needs. Seizures may be controlled with medication and hydrocephalus may require shunting. If feeding becomes difficult, a gastrostomy tube may be considered.

The prognosis for children with lissencephaly varies depending on the degree of brain malformation. Many individuals show no significant development beyond a 3- to 5-month-old level. Some may have near-normal development and intelligence. Many will die before the age of 2. Respiratory problems are the most common causes of death.

Megalencephaly

Megalencephaly, also called macrencephaly, is a condition in which there is an abnormally large, heavy, and usually malfunctioning brain. By definition, the brain weight is greater than average for the age and gender of the infant or child. Head enlargement may be evident at birth or the head may become abnormally large in the early years of life.

Megalencephaly is thought to be related to a disturbance in the regulation of cell reproduction or proliferation. In normal development, neuron proliferation - the process in which nerve cells divide to form new generations of cells - is regulated so that the correct number of cells is formed in the proper place at the appropriate time.

Symptoms of megalencephaly may include delayed development, convulsive disorders, corticospinal (brain cortex and spinal cord) dysfunction, and seizures. Megalencephaly affects males more often than females.

The prognosis for individuals with megalencephaly largely depends on the underlying cause and the associated neurological disorders. Treatment is symptomatic. Megalencephaly may lead to a condition called macrocephaly (defined later in this fact sheet). Unilateral megalencephaly or hemimegalencephaly is a rare condition characterized by the enlargement of one-half of the brain. Children with this disorder may have a large, sometimes asymmetrical head. Often they suffer from intractable seizures and mental retardation. The prognosis for those with hemimegalencephaly is poor.

Microcephaly

Microcephaly is a neurological disorder in which the circumference of the head is smaller than average for the age and gender of the infant or child. Microcephaly may be congenital or it may develop in the first few years of life. The disorder may stem from a wide variety of conditions that cause abnormal growth of the brain, or from syndromes associated with chromosomal abnormalities.

Infants with microcephaly are born with either a normal or reduced head size. Subsequently the head fails to grow while the face continues to develop at a normal rate, producing a child with a small head, a large face, a receding forehead, and a loose, often wrinkled scalp. As the child grows older, the smallness of the skull becomes more obvious, although the entire body also is often underweight and dwarfed. Development of motor functions and speech may be delayed. Hyperactivity and mental retardation are common occurrences, although the degree of each varies. Convulsions may also occur. Motor ability varies, ranging from clumsiness in some to spastic quadriplegia in others.

Generally there is no specific treatment for microcephaly. Treatment is symptomatic and supportive.

In general, life expectancy for individuals with microcephaly is reduced and the prognosis for normal brain function is poor. The prognosis varies depending on the presence of associated abnormalities.

Porencephaly

Porencephaly is an extremely rare disorder of the central nervous system involving a cyst or cavity in a cerebral hemisphere. The cysts or cavities are usually the remnants of destructive lesions, but are sometimes the result of abnormal development. The disorder can occur before or after birth.

Porencephaly most likely has a number of different, often unknown causes, including absence of brain development and destruction of brain tissue. The presence of porencephalic cysts can sometimes be detected by transillumination of the skull in infancy. The diagnosis may be confirmed by CT, MRI, or ultrasonography.

More severely affected infants show symptoms of the disorder shortly after birth, and the diagnosis is usually made before age 1. Signs may include delayed growth and development, spastic paresis (slight or incomplete paralysis), hypotonia (decreased muscle tone), seizures (often infantile spasms), and macrocephaly or microcephaly.

Individuals with porencephaly may have poor or absent speech development, epilepsy, hydrocephalus, spastic contractures (shrinkage or shortening of muscles), and mental retardation. Treatment may include physical therapy, medication for seizure disorders, and a shunt for hydrocephalus. The prognosis for individuals with porencephaly varies according to the location and extent of the lesion. Some patients with this disorder may develop only minor neurological problems and have normal intelligence, while others may be severely disabled. Others may die before the second decade of life.

Schizencephaly

Schizencephaly is a rare developmental disorder characterized by abnormal slits, or clefts, in the cerebral hemispheres. Schizencephaly is a form of porencephaly. Individuals with clefts in both hemispheres, or bilateral clefts, are often developmentally delayed and have delayed speech and language skills and corticospinal dysfunction. Individuals with smaller, unilateral clefts (clefts in one hemisphere) may be weak on one side of the body and may have average or near-average intelligence. Patients with schizencephaly may also have varying degrees of microcephaly, mental retardation, hemiparesis (weakness or paralysis affecting one side of the body), or quadriparesis (weakness or paralysis affecting all four extremities), and may have reduced muscle tone (hypotonia). Most patients have seizures and some may have hydrocephalus.

In schizencephaly, the neurons border the edge of the cleft implying a very early disruption in development. There is now a genetic origin for one type of schizencephaly. Causes of this type may include environmental exposures during pregnancy such as medication taken by the mother, exposure to toxins, or a vascular insult. Often there are associated heterotopias (isolated islands of neurons) which indicate a failure of migration of the neurons to their final position in the brain.

Treatment for individuals with schizencephaly generally consists of physical therapy, treatment for seizures, and, in cases that are complicated by hydrocephalus, a shunt.

The prognosis for individuals with schizencephaly varies depending on the size of the clefts and the degree of neurological deficit.

Less Common Cephalies

Acephaly

Acephaly literally means absence of the head. It is a much rarer condition than anencephaly. The acephalic fetus is a parasitic twin attached to an otherwise intact fetus. The acephalic fetus has a body but lacks a head and a heart; the fetus's neck is attached to the normal twin. The blood circulation of the acephalic fetus is provided by the heart of the twin. The acephalic fetus cannot exist independently of the fetus to which it is attached.

Exencephaly

Exencephaly is a condition in which the brain is located outside of the skull. This condition is usually found in embryos as an early stage of anencephaly. As an exencephalic pregnancy progresses, the neural tissue gradually degenerates. It is unusual to find an infant carried to term with this condition because the defect is incompatible with survival.

Macrocephaly

Macrocephaly is a condition in which the head circumference is larger than average for the age and gender of the infant or child. It is a descriptive rather than a diagnostic term, and is a characteristic of a variety of disorders. Macrocephaly also may be inherited. Although one form of macrocephaly may be associated with mental retardation, in approximately one-half of cases mental development is normal. Macrocephaly may be caused by an enlarged brain or hydrocephalus. It may be associated with other disorders such as dwarfism, neurofibromatosis, and tuberous sclerosis.

Micrencephaly

Micrencephaly is a disorder characterized by a small brain and may be caused by a disturbance in the proliferation of nerve cells. Micrencephaly may also be associated with maternal problems such as alcoholism, diabetes, or rubella (German measles). A genetic factor may play a role in causing some cases of micrencephaly. Affected newborns generally have striking neurological defects and seizures. Severely impaired intellectual development is common, but disturbances in motor functions may not appear until later in life.

Octocephaly

Octocephaly is a lethal condition in which the primary feature is agnathia - a developmental anomaly characterized by total or virtual absence of the lower jaw. The condition is considered lethal because of a poorly functioning airway. In octocephaly, agnathia may occur alone or together with holoprosencephaly.

Another group of less common cephalic disorders are the craniostenoses. Craniostenoses are deformities of the skull caused by the premature fusion or joining together of the cranial sutures. Cranial sutures are fibrous joints that join the bones of the skull together. The nature of these deformities depends on which sutures are affected.

Brachycephaly

Brachycephaly occurs when the coronal suture fuses prematurely, causing a shortened front-to-back diameter of the skull. The coronal suture is the fibrous joint that unites the frontal bone with the two parietal bones of the skull. The parietal bones form the top and sides of the skull.

Oxycephaly

Oxycephaly is a term sometimes used to describe the premature closure of the coronal suture plus any other suture, or it may be used to describe the premature fusing of all sutures. Oxycephaly is the most severe of the craniostenoses.

Plagiocephaly

Plagiocephaly results from the premature unilateral fusion (joining of one side) of the coronal or lambdoid sutures. The lambdoid suture unites the occipital bone with the parietal bones of the skull. Plagiocephaly is a condition characterized by an asymmetrical distortion (flattening of one side) of the skull. It is a common finding at birth and may be the result of brain malformation, a restrictive intrauterine environment, or torticollis (a spasm or tightening of neck muscles).

Scaphocephaly

Scaphocephaly applies to premature fusion of the sagittal suture. The sagittal suture joins together the two parietal bones of skull. Scaphocephaly is the most common of the craniostenoses and is characterized by a long, narrow head.

Trigonocephaly

Trigonocephaly is the premature fusion of the metopic suture (part of the frontal suture which joins the two halves of the frontal bone of the skull) in which a V-shaped abnormality occurs at the front of the skull. It is characterized by the triangular prominence of the forehead and closely set eyes.

What Research Is Being Done?

Within the Federal Government, the National Institute of Neurological Disorders and Stroke (NINDS), one of the National Institutes of Health (NIH), has primary responsibility for conducting and supporting research on normal and abnormal brain and nervous system development, including congenital anomalies. The National Institute of Child Health and Human Development, the National Institute of Mental Health, the National Institute of Environmental Health Sciences, the National Institute of Alcohol Abuse and Alcoholism, and the National Institute on Drug Abuse also support research related to disorders of the developing nervous system. Gaining basic knowledge about how the nervous system develops and understanding the role of genetics in fetal development are major goals of scientists studying congenital neurological disorders.

Scientists are rapidly learning how harmful insults at various stages of pregnancy can lead to developmental disorders. For example, a critical nutritional deficiency or exposure to an environmental insult during the first month of pregnancy (when the neural tube is formed) can produce neural tube defects such as anencephaly.

Scientists are also concentrating their efforts on understanding the complex processes responsible for normal early development of the brain and nervous system and how the disruption of any of these processes results in congenital anomalies such as cephalic disorders. Recently, two new genes have been discovered that are causes of lissencephaly and milder neuronal migration disorders. Understanding how genes control brain cell migration, proliferation, differentiation, and death, and how radiation, drugs, toxins, infections, and other factors disrupt these processes will aid in preventing many congenital neurological disorders.

Currently, researchers are examining the mechanisms involved in neurulation - the process of forming the neural tube. These studies will improve our understanding of this process and give insight into how the process can go awry and cause devastating congenital disorders.

Investigators are also conducting a variety of genetic studies. One of these studies concentrates on a specific form of holoprosencephaly with the goal of finding the basic DNA defect responsible for the abnormal development seen in this disorder. Researchers are also analyzing genes and gene products necessary for human brain development to achieve a better understanding of normal brain development in humans.

Other research projects currently under way include a study to evaluate increased risk of neural tube defects and various other congenital malformations in association with environmental and occupational exposure to pesticides.

Where Can I Go for More Information?

For more information about disorders of the developing nervous system, cephalic disorders, or birth defects in general, you may wish to contact:

National Organization for Rare Disorders (NORD)
P.O. Box 8923
New Fairfield, Connecticut 06812-8923
(203) 746-6518
(800) 999-6673
www.rarediseases.org

The Lissencephaly Network, Inc.
716 Autumn Ridge Lane
Fort Wayne, Indiana 46804-6402
(219) 432-4310
www.lissencephaly.org

The March of Dimes Birth Defects Foundation
1275 Mamaroneck Avenue
White Plains, New York 10605
(914) 428-7100
(888) MODIMES (663-4637)
www.modimes.org

Association of Birth Defects Children
930 Woodcock Rd.

Orlando, Florida 32803
(407) 245-7035
(800) 313-ABDC (2232)
www.birthdefects.org

For more information on research on the cephalic disorders, you may wish to contact the NINDS Brain Resources and Information Network (BRAIN) at:

BRAIN
P.O. Box 5801
Bethesda, MD 20824
(800) 352-9424
http://www.ninds.nih.gov

In addition the general guideline above, the NINDS has recently published the following guideline:

What Is Megalencephaly?[8]

Megalencephaly, also called macrencephaly, is a condition in which there is an abnormally large, heavy, and usually malfunctioning brain. By definition, the brain weight is greater than average for the age and gender of the individual. Head enlargement may be evident at birth or the head may become abnormally large in the early years of life. Megalencephaly is thought to be related to a disturbance in the regulation of cell reproduction or proliferation. In normal development, neuron proliferation - the process in which nerve cells divide to form new generations of cells - is regulated so that the correct number of cells is formed in the proper place at the appropriate time. Symptoms of megalencephaly may include delayed development, convulsive disorders, corticospinal (brain cortex and spinal cord) dysfunction, and seizures. Megalencephaly affects males more often than females. Unilateral megalencephaly or hemimegalencephaly is a rare condition and is characterized by the enlargement of one-half of the brain. Children with this disorder may have a large, sometimes asymmetrical head. Often they suffer from intractable seizures and mental retardation.

[8] Adapted from The National Institute of Neurological Disorders and Stroke (NINDS): **http://www.ninds.nih.gov/health_and_medical/disorders/megalencephaly.htm**.

Is There Any Treatment?

There is no definitive treatment for megalencephaly. Treatment is symptomatic and supportive.

What Is the Prognosis?

The prognosis for individuals with megalencephaly largely depends on the underlying cause and the associated neurological disorders. The prognosis for those with hemimegalencephaly is poor.

What Research Is Being Done?

The NINDS supports and conducts neurogenetic research which focuses on identifying and studying the genes involved in normal brain development. The knowledge gained from these fundamental studies provides the foundation for understanding how this process can go awry and, thus, may eventually give clues to understanding disorders such as megalencephaly.

Selected References

Bradley, W, et al (eds).
Neurology in Clinical Practice: The Neurological Disorders. vol. II, 2nd edition, Butterworth-Heinemann, Boston, p. 1480 (1996).

Rowland, L (ed).
Merritt's Textbook of Neurology. 9th edition, Williams & Wilkins, Baltimore, pp. 519-520 (1995).

Asbury, A, et. al. (eds).
Diseases of the Nervous System: Clinical Neurobiology. vol. I, 2nd edition, W.B. Saunders Co., Philadelphia, pp. 616-617 (1992).

Gooskens, R, et. al.
Megalencephaly: Definition and Classification. Brain & Development, 10:1; 1-7 (1988).

DeMyer, W.
Megalencephaly: Types, Clinical Syndromes, and Management. Pediatric Neurology, 2:6; 321-328 (1986).

For More Information

For more information, contact:

March of Dimes Birth Defects Foundation
1275 Mamaroneck Avenue
White Plains, NY 10605
resourcecenter@modimes.org
http://www.modimes.org
Tel: 914-428-7100 / 888-MODIMES (663-4637)
Fax: 914-428-8203

National Organization for Rare Disorders (NORD)
P.O. Box 8923
(100 Route 37)
New Fairfield, CT 06812-8923
orphan@rarediseases.org
http://www.rarediseases.org
Tel: 203-746-6518 / 800-999-NORD (6673)
Fax: 203-746-6481

National Institute of Child Health and Human Development (NICHD)
National Institutes of Health
Bldg. 31, Rm. 2A32
Bethesda, MD 20892-2425
NICHDClearinghouse@mail.nih.gov
http://www.nichd.nih.gov
Tel: 301-496-5133 / 800-370-2943

More Guideline Sources

The guideline above on megalencephaly is only one example of the kind of material that you can find online and free of charge. The remainder of this chapter will direct you to other sources which either publish or can help you find additional guidelines on topics related to megalencephaly. Many of the guidelines listed below address topics that may be of particular relevance to your child's specific situation, while certain guidelines will apply to only some children with megalencephaly. Due to space limitations these sources are listed in a concise manner. Do not hesitate to consult the following sources by either using the Internet hyperlink provided, or, in cases where the contact information is provided, contacting the publisher or author directly.

Topic Pages: MEDLINEplus

For parents wishing to go beyond guidelines published by specific Institutes of the NIH, the National Library of Medicine has created a vast and parent-oriented healthcare information portal called MEDLINEplus. Within this Internet-based system are "health topic pages." You can think of a health topic page as a guide to patient guides. To access this system, log on to **http://www.nlm.nih.gov/medlineplus/healthtopics.html**.

You may also choose to use the search utility provided by MEDLINEplus at the following Web address: **http://www.nlm.nih.gov/medlineplus/**. Simply type a keyword into the search box and click "Search." This utility is similar to the NIH search utility, with the exception that it only includes materials that are linked within the MEDLINEplus system (mostly patient-oriented information). It also has the disadvantage of generating unstructured results. We recommend, therefore, that you use this method only if you have a very targeted search.

The National Guideline Clearinghouse™

The National Guideline Clearinghouse™ offers hundreds of evidence-based clinical practice guidelines published in the United States and other countries. You can search their site located at **http://www.guideline.gov** by using the keyword "megalencephaly" or synonyms.

The NIH Search Utility

After browsing the references listed at the beginning of this chapter, you may want to explore the NIH search utility. This allows you to search for documents on over 100 selected Web sites that comprise the NIH-WEB-SPACE. Each of these servers is "crawled" and indexed on an ongoing basis. Your search will produce a list of various documents, all of which will relate in some way to megalencephaly. The drawbacks of this approach are that the information is not organized by theme and that the references are often a mix of information for professionals and parents. Nevertheless, a large number of the listed Web sites provide useful background information. We can only recommend this route, therefore, for relatively rare or specific disorders, or when using highly targeted searches. To use the NIH search utility, visit the following Web page: **http://search.nih.gov/index.html**.

Additional Web Sources

A number of Web sites that often link to government sites are available to the public. These can also point you in the direction of essential information. The following is a representative sample:

- AOL: **http://search.aol.com/cat.adp?id=168&layer=&from=subcats**
- Family Village: **http://www.familyvillage.wisc.edu/specific.htm**
- Google: **http://directory.google.com/Top/Health/Conditions_and_Diseases/**
- Med Help International: **http://www.medhelp.org/HealthTopics/A.html**
- Open Directory Project: **http://dmoz.org/Health/Conditions_and_Diseases/**
- Yahoo.com: **http://dir.yahoo.com/Health/Diseases_and_Conditions/**
- WebMD®Health: **http://my.webmd.com/health_topics**

Vocabulary Builder

The material in this chapter may have contained a number of unfamiliar words. The following Vocabulary Builder introduces you to terms used in this chapter that have not been covered in the previous chapter:

Anticonvulsant: An agent that prevents or relieves convulsions. [EU]

Bilateral: Having two sides, or pertaining to both sides. [EU]

Cardiovascular: Pertaining to the heart and blood vessels. [EU]

Cerebellum: Part of the metencephalon that lies in the posterior cranial fossa behind the brain stem. It is concerned with the coordination of movement. [NIH]

Cerebral: Of or pertaining of the cerebrum or the brain. [EU]

Cerebrospinal: Pertaining to the brain and spinal cord. [EU]

Chromosomal: Pertaining to chromosomes. [EU]

Chronic: Persisting over a long period of time. [EU]

Consciousness: Sense of awareness of self and of the environment. [NIH]

Contracture: A condition of fixed high resistance to passive stretch of a muscle, resulting from fibrosis of the tissues supporting the muscles or the joints, or from disorders of the muscle fibres. [EU]

Convulsion: A violent involuntary contraction or series of contractions of the voluntary muscles. [EU]

Cortex: The outer layer of an organ or other body structure, as distinguished from the internal substance. [EU]

Cranial: Pertaining to the cranium, or to the anterior (in animals) or superior (in humans) end of the body. [EU]

Cyst: Any closed cavity or sac; normal or abnormal, lined by epithelium, and especially one that contains a liquid or semisolid material. [EU]

Embryo: In animals, those derivatives of the fertilized ovum that eventually become the offspring, during their period of most rapid development, i.e., after the long axis appears until all major structures are represented. In man, the developing organism is an embryo from about two weeks after fertilization to the end of seventh or eighth week. [EU]

Facial: Of or pertaining to the face. [EU]

Gastrointestinal: Pertaining to or communicating with the stomach and intestine, as a gastrointestinal fistula. [EU]

Gastrostomy: Creation of an artificial external opening into the stomach for nutritional support or gastrointestinal compression. [NIH]

Hernia: (he protrusion of a loop or knuckle of an organ or tissue through an abnormal opening. [EU]

Hydrocephalus: A condition marked by dilatation of the cerebral ventricles, most often occurring secondarily to obstruction of the cerebrospinal fluid pathways, and accompanied by an accumulation of cerebrospinal fluid within the skull; the fluid is usually under increased pressure, but occasionally may be normal or nearly so. It is typically characterized by enlargement of the head, prominence of the forehead, brain atrophy, mental deterioration, and convulsions; may be congenital or acquired; and may be of sudden onset (acute h.) or be slowly progressive (chronic or primary b.). [EU]

Hypertonia: Or hypertony n, pl. hypertonias or hypertonies : hypertonicity. n. Pathology: increased rigidity, tension and spasticity of the muscles. [EU]

Hypotonia: A condition of diminished tone of the skeletal muscles; diminished resistance of muscles to passive stretching. [EU]

Infantile: Pertaining to an infant or to infancy. [EU]

Lesion: Any pathological or traumatic discontinuity of tissue or loss of function of a part. [EU]

Lethal: Deadly, fatal. [EU]

Lip: Either of the two fleshy, full-blooded margins of the mouth. [NIH]

Malformation: A morphologic defect resulting from an intrinsically abnormal developmental process. [EU]

Mandible: The largest and strongest bone of the FACE constituting the lower jaw. It supports the lower teeth. [NIH]

Neural: 1. Pertaining to a nerve or to the nerves. 2. Situated in the region of the spinal axis, as the neutral arch. [EU]

Neurology: A medical specialty concerned with the study of the structures, functions, and diseases of the nervous system. [NIH]

Neuronal: Pertaining to a neuron or neurons (= conducting cells of the nervous system). [EU]

Neurons: The basic cellular units of nervous tissue. Each neuron consists of a body, an axon, and dendrites. Their purpose is to receive, conduct, and transmit impulses in the nervous system. [NIH]

Paralysis: Loss or impairment of motor function in a part due to lesion of the neural or muscular mechanism; also by analogy, impairment of sensory function (sensory paralysis). In addition to the types named below, paralysis is further distinguished as traumatic, syphilitic, toxic, etc., according to its cause; or as obturator, ulnar, etc., according to the nerve part, or muscle specially affected. [EU]

Parasitic: Pertaining to, of the nature of, or caused by a parasite. [EU]

Parietal: 1. Of or pertaining to the walls of a cavity. 2. Pertaining to or located near the parietal bone, as the parietal lobe. [EU]

Posterior: Situated in back of, or in the back part of, or affecting the back or dorsal surface of the body. In lower animals, it refers to the caudal end of the body. [EU]

Prosencephalon: The part of the brain developed from the most rostral of the three primary vesicles of the embryonic neural tube and consisting of the diencephalon and telencephalon. [NIH]

Psychomotor: Pertaining to motor effects of cerebral or psychic activity. [EU]

Quadriplegia: Severe or complete loss of motor function in all four limbs which may result from brain diseases; spinal cord diseases; peripheral nervous system diseases; neuromuscular diseases; or rarely muscular diseases. The locked-in syndrome is characterized by quadriplegia in combination with cranial muscle paralysis. Consciousness is spared and the only retained voluntary motor activity may be limited eye movements. This condition is usually caused by a lesion in the upper BRAIN STEM which injures the descending cortico-spinal and cortico-bulbar tracts. [NIH]

Reflex: 1. Reflected. 2. A reflected action or movement; the sum total of any particular involuntary activity. [EU]

Rubella: An acute, usually benign, infectious disease caused by a togavirus and most often affecting children and nonimmune young adults, in which the virus enters the respiratory tract via droplet nuclei and spreads to the lymphatic system. It is characterized by a slight cold, sore throat, and fever, followed by enlargement of the postauricular, suboccipital, and cervical lymph nodes, and the appearances of a fine pink rash that begins on the head and spreads to become generalized. Called also German measles, roetln, röteln, and three-day measles, and rubeola in French and Spanish. [EU]

Sclerosis: A induration, or hardening; especially hardening of a part from inflammation and in diseases of the interstitial substance. The term is used chiefly for such a hardening of the nervous system due to hyperplasia of the connective tissue or to designate hardening of the blood vessels. [EU]

Seizures: Clinical or subclinical disturbances of cortical function due to a sudden, abnormal, excessive, and disorganized discharge of brain cells. Clinical manifestations include abnormal motor, sensory and psychic phenomena. Recurrent seizures are usually referred to as epilepsy or "seizure disorder." [NIH]

Shunt: 1. To turn to one side; to divert; to bypass. 2. A passage or anastomosis between two natural channels, especially between blood vessels. Such structures may be formed physiologically (e.g. to bypass a thrombosis) or they may be structural anomalies. 3. a surgically created anastomosis; also, the operation of forming a shunt. [EU]

Skull: The skeleton of the head including the bones of the face and the bones enclosing the brain. [NIH]

Spastic: 1. Of the nature of or characterized by spasms. 2. Hypertonic, so that the muscles are stiff and the movements awkward. 3. A person exhibiting spasticity, such as occurs in spastic paralysis or in cerebral palsy. [EU]

Spectrum: A charted band of wavelengths of electromagnetic vibrations obtained by refraction and diffraction. By extension, a measurable range of activity, such as the range of bacteria affected by an antibiotic (antibacterial s.) or the complete range of manifestations of a disease. [EU]

Symptomatic: 1. Pertaining to or of the nature of a symptom. 2. Indicative (of a particular disease or disorder). 3. Exhibiting the symptoms of a particular disease but having a different cause. 4. Directed at the allying of symptoms, as symptomatic treatment. [EU]

Tomography: The recording of internal body images at a predetermined plane by means of the tomograph; called also body section roentgenography.

[EU]

Tone: 1. The normal degree of vigour and tension; in muscle, the resistance to passive elongation or stretch; tonus. 2. A particular quality of sound or of voice. 3. To make permanent, or to change, the color of silver stain by chemical treatment, usually with a heavy metal. [EU]

Torticollis: Wryneck; a contracted state of the cervical muscles, producing twisting of the neck and an unnatural position of the head. [EU]

Toxin: A poison; frequently used to refer specifically to a protein produced by some higher plants, certain animals, and pathogenic bacteria, which is highly toxic for other living organisms. Such substances are differentiated from the simple chemical poisons and the vegetable alkaloids by their high molecular weight and antigenicity. [EU]

Transillumination: Passage of light through body tissues or cavities for examination of internal structures. [NIH]

Trisomy: The possession of a third chromosome of any one type in an otherwise diploid cell. [NIH]

Ultrasonography: The visualization of deep structures of the body by recording the reflections of echoes of pulses of ultrasonic waves directed into the tissues. Use of ultrasound for imaging or diagnostic purposes employs frequencies ranging from 1.6 to 10 megahertz. [NIH]

Vascular: Pertaining to blood vessels or indicative of a copious blood supply. [EU]

Viral: Pertaining to, caused by, or of the nature of virus. [EU]

CHAPTER 2. SEEKING GUIDANCE

Overview

Some parents are comforted by the knowledge that a number of organizations dedicate their resources to helping people with megalencephaly. These associations can become invaluable sources of information and advice. Many associations offer parent support, financial assistance, and other important services. Furthermore, healthcare research has shown that support groups often help people to better cope with their conditions.[9] In addition to support groups, your child's physician can be a valuable source of guidance and support.

In this chapter, we direct you to resources that can help you find parent organizations and medical specialists. We begin by describing how to find associations and parent groups that can help you better understand and cope with your child's condition. The chapter ends with a discussion on how to find a doctor that is right for your child.

Finding Associations

There are several Internet directories that provide lists of medical associations with information on or resources relating to megalencephaly. By consulting all of associations listed in this chapter, you will have nearly exhausted all sources for parent associations concerned with megalencephaly.

---

[9] Churches, synagogues, and other houses of worship might also have groups that can offer you the social support you need.

The National Health Information Center (NHIC)

The National Health Information Center (NHIC) offers a free referral service to help people find organizations that provide information about megalencephaly. For more information, see the NHIC's Web site at **http://www.health.gov/NHIC/** or contact an information specialist by calling 1-800-336-4797.

DIRLINE

A comprehensive source of information on associations is the DIRLINE database maintained by the National Library of Medicine. The database comprises some 10,000 records of organizations, research centers, and government institutes and associations which primarily focus on health and biomedicine. DIRLINE is available via the Internet at the following Web site: **http://dirline.nlm.nih.gov**. Simply type in "megalencephaly" (or a synonym) or the name of a topic, and the site will list information contained in the database on all relevant organizations.

The Combined Health Information Database

Another comprehensive source of information on healthcare associations is the Combined Health Information Database. Using the "Detailed Search" option, you will need to limit your search to "Organizations" and "megalencephaly". Type the following hyperlink into your Web browser: **http://chid.nih.gov/detail/detail.html**. To find associations, use the drop boxes at the bottom of the search page where "You may refine your search by." For publication date, select "All Years." Then, select your preferred language and the format option "Organization Resource Sheet." By making these selections and typing in "megalencephaly" (or synonyms) into the "For these words:" box, you will only receive results on organizations dealing with megalencephaly. You should check back periodically with this database since it is updated every 3 months.

The National Organization for Rare Disorders, Inc.

The National Organization for Rare Disorders, Inc. has prepared a Web site that provides, at no charge, lists of associations organized by specific medical conditions. You can access this database at the following Web site:

http://www.rarediseases.org/search/orgsearch.html. Type "megalencephaly" (or a synonym) in the search box, and click "Submit Query."

Online Support Groups

In addition to support groups, commercial Internet service providers offer forums and chat rooms to discuss different illnesses and conditions. WebMD®, for example, offers such a service at its Web site: **http://boards.webmd.com/roundtable**. These online communities can help you connect with a network of people whose concerns are similar to yours. Online support groups are places where people can talk informally. If you read about a novel approach, consult with your child's doctor or other healthcare providers, as the treatments or discoveries you hear about may not be scientifically proven to be safe and effective.

Finding Doctors

All parents must go through the process of selecting a physician for their children with megalencephaly. While this process will vary, the Agency for Healthcare Research and Quality makes a number of suggestions, including the following:[10]

- If your child is in a managed care plan, check the plan's list of doctors first.
- Ask doctors or other health professionals who work with doctors, such as hospital nurses, for referrals.
- Call a hospital's doctor referral service, but keep in mind that these services usually refer you to doctors on staff at that particular hospital. The services do not have information on the quality of care that these doctors provide.
- Some local medical societies offer lists of member doctors. Again, these lists do not have information on the quality of care that these doctors provide.

Additional steps you can take to locate doctors include the following:

- Check with the associations listed earlier in this chapter.

---

[10] This section has been adapted from the AHRQ: **www.ahrq.gov/consumer/qntascii/qntdr.htm**.

- Information on doctors in some states is available on the Internet at **http://www.docboard.org**. This Web site is run by "Administrators in Medicine," a group of state medical board directors.
- The American Board of Medical Specialties can tell you if your child's doctor is board certified. "Certified" means that the doctor has completed a training program in a specialty and has passed an exam, or "board," to assess his or her knowledge, skills, and experience to provide quality patient care in that specialty. Primary care doctors may also be certified as specialists. The AMBS Web site is located at **http://www.abms.org/newsearch.asp**.[11] You can also contact the ABMS by phone at 1-866-ASK-ABMS.
- You can call the American Medical Association (AMA) at 800-665-2882 for information on training, specialties, and board certification for many licensed doctors in the United States. This information also can be found in "Physician Select" at the AMA's Web site: **http://www.ama-assn.org/aps/amahg.htm**.

Finding a Neurologist

The American Academy of Neurology allows you to search for member neurologists by name or location. To use this service, go to **http://www.aan.com/**, select "Find a Neurologist" from the toolbar. Enter your search criteria, and click "Search." To find out more information on a particular neurologist, click on the physician's name.

If the previous sources did not meet your needs, you may want to log on to the Web site of the National Organization for Rare Disorders (NORD) at **http://www.rarediseases.org/**. NORD maintains a database of doctors with expertise in various rare diseases. The Metabolic Information Network (MIN), 800-945-2188, also maintains a database of physicians with expertise in various metabolic diseases.

Selecting Your Child's Doctor[12]

When you have compiled a list of prospective doctors, call each of their offices. First, ask if the doctor accepts your child's health insurance plan and

---

[11] While board certification is a good measure of a doctor's knowledge, it is possible to receive quality care from doctors who are not board certified.

[12] This section has been adapted from the AHRQ: **www.ahrq.gov/consumer/qntascii/qntdr.htm**.

if he or she is taking new patients. If the doctor is not covered by your child's plan, ask yourself if you are prepared to pay the extra costs. The next step is to schedule a visit with your first choice. During the first visit you will have the opportunity to evaluate your child's doctor and to find out if your child feels comfortable with him or her.

Working with Your Child's Doctor[13]

Research has shown that parents who have good relationships with their children's doctors tend to be more satisfied with their children's care. Here are some tips to help you and your child's doctor become partners:

- You know important things about your child's symptoms and health history. Tell the doctor what you think he or she needs to know.
- Always bring any medications your child is currently taking with you to the appointment, or you can bring a list of your child's medications including dosage and frequency information. Talk about any allergies or reactions your child has had to medications.
- Tell your doctor about any natural or alternative medicines your child is taking.
- Bring other medical information, such as x-ray films, test results, and medical records.
- Ask questions. If you don't, the doctor will assume that you understood everything that was said.
- Write down your questions before the doctor's visit. List the most important ones first to make sure that they are addressed.
- Ask the doctor to draw pictures if you think that this will help you and your child understand.
- Take notes. Some doctors do not mind if you bring a tape recorder to help you remember things, but always ask first.
- Take information home. Ask for written instructions. Your child's doctor may also have brochures and audio and videotapes on megalencephaly.

By following these steps, you will enhance the relationship you and your child have with the physician.

---

[13] This section has been adapted from the AHRQ: **www.ahrq.gov/consumer/qntascii/qntdr.htm**.

Broader Health-Related Resources

In addition to the references above, the NIH has set up guidance Web sites that can help parents find healthcare professionals. These include:[14]

- Caregivers: **http://www.nlm.nih.gov/medlineplus/caregivers.html**
- Choosing a Doctor or Healthcare Service: **http://www.nlm.nih.gov/medlineplus/choosingadoctororhealthcareservice.html**
- Hospitals and Health Facilities: **http://www.nlm.nih.gov/medlineplus/healthfacilities.html**

[14] You can access this information at **http://www.nlm.nih.gov/medlineplus/healthsystem.html**.

PART II: ADDITIONAL RESOURCES AND ADVANCED MATERIAL

ABOUT PART II

In Part II, we introduce you to additional resources and advanced research on megalencephaly. All too often, parents who conduct their own research are overwhelmed by the difficulty in finding and organizing information. The purpose of the following chapters is to provide you an organized and structured format to help you find additional information resources on megalencephaly. In Part II, as in Part I, our objective is not to interpret the latest advances on megalencephaly or render an opinion. Rather, our goal is to give you access to original research and to increase your awareness of sources you may not have already considered. In this way, you will come across the advanced materials often referred to in pamphlets, books, or other general works. Once again, some of this material is technical in nature, so consultation with a professional familiar with megalencephaly is suggested.

CHAPTER 3. STUDIES ON MEGALENCEPHALY

Overview

Every year, academic studies are published on megalencephaly or related conditions. Broadly speaking, there are two types of studies. The first are peer reviewed. Generally, the content of these studies has been reviewed by scientists or physicians. Peer-reviewed studies are typically published in scientific journals and are usually available at medical libraries. The second type of studies is non-peer reviewed. These works include summary articles that do not use or report scientific results. These often appear in the popular press, newsletters, or similar periodicals.

In this chapter, we will show you how to locate peer-reviewed references and studies on megalencephaly. We will begin by discussing research that has been summarized and is free to view by the public via the Internet. We then show you how to generate a bibliography on megalencephaly and teach you how to keep current on new studies as they are published or undertaken by the scientific community.

The Combined Health Information Database

The Combined Health Information Database summarizes studies across numerous federal agencies. To limit your investigation to research studies and megalencephaly, you will need to use the advanced search options. First, go to **http://chid.nih.gov/index.html**. From there, select the "Detailed Search" option (or go directly to that page with the following hyperlink: **http://chid.nih.gov/detail/detail.html**). The trick in extracting studies is found in the drop boxes at the bottom of the search page where "You may refine your search by." Select the dates and language you prefer, and the format option "Journal Article." At the top of the search form, select the number of records you would like to see (we recommend 100) and check the box to display "whole records." We recommend that you type in "megalencephaly" (or synonyms) into the "For these words:" box. Consider using the option "anywhere in record" to make your search as broad as possible. If you want to limit the search to only a particular field, such as the title of the journal, then select this option in the "Search in these fields" drop box. The following is a sample of what you can expect from this type of search:

- **Canavan Disease: An Expanded Role for Dentists**

  Source: SCD. Special Care in Dentistry. 18(3): 119-122. May-June 1998.

  Contact: Available from Special Care Dentistry. 211 East Chicago Avenue, Chicago, IL 60611. (312) 440-2660. Fax (312) 440-2824.

  Summary: Canavan disease (CD) is a progressive neurodegenerative disease that occurs predominantly but not exclusively in Ashkenazi Jews. It is characterized by a normal birth, rapidly followed by signs of lack of interest, hypotonia, and **megalencephaly**, resulting in early death. Death was initially believed to occur before the age of three years; however, some individuals have survived into their teenage years. Recent studies suggest that there may be a separate, more protracted type of CD. A long life expectancy necessitates the rendering of dental treatment for these children, whose oral health in the past may have been neglected due to their short life expectancy. This article reviews the disease and the role of the dentist in the treatment of infants and children afflicted with this disorder. The authors note that early dental treatment may support parents and siblings in caring for the child with CD and help create good family dynamics. 3 figures. 25 references. (AA-M).

Federally Funded Research on Megalencephaly

The U.S. Government supports a variety of research studies relating to megalencephaly and associated conditions. These studies are tracked by the Office of Extramural Research at the National Institutes of Health.[15] CRISP (Computerized Retrieval of Information on Scientific Projects) is a searchable database of federally funded biomedical research projects conducted at

[15] Healthcare projects are funded by the National Institutes of Health (NIH), Substance Abuse and Mental Health Services (SAMHSA), Health Resources and Services Administration (HRSA), Food and Drug Administration (FDA), Centers for Disease Control and Prevention (CDCP), Agency for Healthcare Research and Quality (AHRQ), and Office of Assistant Secretary of Health (OASH).

universities, hospitals, and other institutions. Visit CRISP at **http://crisp.cit.nih.gov/crisp/crisp_query.generate_screen**. You can perform targeted searches by various criteria including geography, date, as well as topics related to megalencephaly and related conditions.

For most of the studies, the agencies reporting into CRISP provide summaries or abstracts. As opposed to clinical trial research using patients, many federally funded studies use animals or simulated models to explore megalencephaly and related conditions. In some cases, therefore, it may be difficult to understand how some basic or fundamental research could eventually translate into medical practice. The following sample is typical of the type of information found when searching the CRISP database for megalencephaly:

- **Project Title: MEGALENCEPHALY IN AUTISM**

  Principal Investigator & Institution: Lainhart, Janet E.; ; University of Utah 200 S University St Salt Lake City, Ut 84112

  Timing: Fiscal Year 2000

  Summary: Results from both our laboratory and others indicate that macrocephaly is present in 14-26% of children and adults with idiopathic autism. MRI studies and post mortem studies of brain weight suggest that macrocephaly in autism is due to megalencephaly, abnormal enlargement of the brain. Results from our laboratory indicate that in autistic individuals unselected for head size, brain size is increased due to increased volume of the parietal, temporal and occipital (i.e., posterior) lobes. Relative to total brain volume the size of the corpus callosum is disproportionately decreased. Additional data suggest that cortical enlargement is predominantly right-sided. MR studies from other centers support the validity of these findings.- Neuropsychological and neurobiological evidence now suggest that autism is a disorder of a complex distributed neural network resulting in anomalous brain organization and connectivity. The finding of megalencephaly in autism suggests that abnormalities of cellular proliferation or programmed cell death are also involved. The overall goal of this application is to build on our previous work in structural imaging and genetics by exploring abnormalities in brain size and shape in autistic individuals with megalencephaly and by examining the significance of these abnormalities for the pathogenesis of this disorder. We propose to: 1) examine anomalous patterns of growth and organization in autistic individuals with megalencephaly as evidenced by abnormalities in the relationship between (a) anterior and posterior cortical brain volume, (b) cortical and corpus callosum size, (c) gray and white matter volume, and, (d) right-

and left-sided cortical lobe volumes; 2) explore developmental mechanisms that may underlie brain enlargement in autism by examining the trajectory of changes in head circumference overtime; 3) examine heterogeneity in the syndrome of autism by exploring the relationship between brain size and shape abnormalities on MRI to clinical features associated with autism including behavioral and neuropsychological characteristics.

Website: **http://crisp.cit.nih.gov/crisp/crisp_query.generate_screen**

The National Library of Medicine: PubMed

One of the quickest and most comprehensive ways to find academic studies in both English and other languages is to use PubMed, maintained by the National Library of Medicine. The advantage of PubMed over previously mentioned sources is that it covers a greater number of domestic and foreign references. It is also free to the public.[16] If the publisher has a Web site that offers full text of its journals, PubMed will provide links to that site, as well as to sites offering other related data. User registration, a subscription fee, or some other type of fee may be required to access the full text of articles in some journals.

To generate your own bibliography of studies dealing with megalencephaly, simply go to the PubMed Web site at **www.ncbi.nlm.nih.gov/pubmed**. Type "megalencephaly" (or synonyms) into the search box, and click "Go."

Vocabulary Builder

Cortical: Pertaining to or of the nature of a cortex or bark. [EU]

Dentists: Individuals licensed to practice dentistry. [NIH]

Idiopathic: Of the nature of an idiopathy; self-originated; of unknown causation. [EU]

Lobe: A more or less well-defined portion of any organ, especially of the brain, lungs, and glands. Lobes are demarcated by fissures, sulci, connective tissue, and by their shape. [EU]

---

[16] PubMed was developed by the National Center for Biotechnology Information (NCBI) at the National Library of Medicine (NLM) at the National Institutes of Health (NIH). The PubMed database was developed in conjunction with publishers of biomedical literature as a search tool for accessing literature citations and linking to full-text journal articles at Web sites of participating publishers. Publishers that participate in PubMed supply NLM with their citations electronically prior to or at the time of publication.

Oral: Pertaining to the mouth, taken through or applied in the mouth, as an oral medication or an oral thermometer. [EU]

Progressive: Advancing; going forward; going from bad to worse; increasing in scope or severity. [EU]

CHAPTER 4. BOOKS ON MEGALENCEPHALY

Overview

This chapter provides bibliographic book references relating to megalencephaly. You have many options to locate books on megalencephaly. The simplest method is to go to your local bookseller and inquire about titles that they have in stock or can special order for you. Some parents, however, prefer online sources (e.g. **www.amazon.com** and **www.bn.com**). In addition to online booksellers, excellent sources for book titles on megalencephaly include the Combined Health Information Database and the National Library of Medicine. Once you have found a title that interests you, visit your local public or medical library to see if it is available for loan.

Chapters on Megalencephaly

Frequently, megalencephaly will be discussed within a book, perhaps within a specific chapter. In order to find chapters that are specifically dealing with megalencephaly, an excellent source of abstracts is the Combined Health Information Database. You will need to limit your search to book chapters and megalencephaly using the "Detailed Search" option. Go directly to the following hyperlink: **http://chid.nih.gov/detail/detail.html**. To find book chapters, use the drop boxes at the bottom of the search page where "You may refine your search by." Select the dates and language you prefer, and the format option "Book Chapter." By making these selections and typing in "megalencephaly" (or synonyms) into the "For these words:" box, you will only receive results on chapters in books. The following is a typical result when searching for book chapters on megalencephaly:

- **Neuropathology of Epilepsy in Adults**

  Source: in Neuropathology of Epilepsy. Scaravilli, F.; ed. Singapore, World Scientific Publishing Co. Pte. Ltd., pp. 339-478, 1998.

  Contact: World Scientific Publishing Co., Inc., 1060 Main Street, Suite 1B, River Edge, NJ 07661. (800) 227-7562. FAX: (888) 977-2665. INTERNET/EMAIL: www.worldscientific.com; wspc@wspc.com.

  Summary: The Neuropathology of Epilepsy in Adults, a chapter in Neuropathology of Epilepsy, provides an overview of the neuropathology of epilepsy in adults. Neuropathological lesions associated with epilepsy in adults are classified as (1) tumors; (2) trauma; (3) vascular disorders; (4) inflammatory and infectious diseases; (5) degenerative and genetic disorders; (6) metabolic disorders; (7) neuronal migration disorders; (8) hamartomas and hamartias; (9) changes secondary to epilepsy; (10) pathological findings in sudden, unexpected death in epilepsy; (11) aging; and (12) hippocampal sclerosis. Tumors include (1) astrocytomas, (2) pilocytic astrocytoma, (3) pleomorphic xanthoastrocytoma, (4) subependymal giant cell gangliocytoma, (5) ganglioglioma and gangliocytoma, and (6) dysembryoplastic neuroepithelial tumor. Types of trauma associated with epilepsy include (1) head contusions and lacerations, (2) intracranial hemorrhage, and (3) hematomas. Cerebrovascular disorders associated with epilepsy include arteriovenous malformations and cavernous angiomas. Inflammatory and infectious diseases associated with epilepsy include (1) vasculitis of the central nervous system, (2) paraneoplastic disorders, and (3) bacterial and viral infections. Degenerative and genetic disorders associated with epilepsy include myoclonus epilepsy and Lafora body disease. Neuronal migration disorders associated with epilepsy include (1) megalencephaly and hemimegalencephaly, (2) defects in gyration, (3) gray matter heterotopias, (4) focal cortical dysplasia, and (5) microdysgenesis. Changes secondary to epilepsy in adults include (1) nerve cell loss, (2) cerebellar atrophy, (3) cerebellar hemiatrophy, (4) contralateral cerebellar atrophy, and (5) changes associated with status epilepticus. Sudden, unexpected death in epilepsy accounts for 5 to 30 percent of epilepsy deaths. The incidence of epilepsy appears to increase significantly after age 60.

General Home References

In addition to references for megalencephaly, you may want a general home medical guide that spans all aspects of home healthcare. The following list is a recent sample of such guides (sorted alphabetically by title; hyperlinks provide rankings, information, and reviews at Amazon.com):

- **Adams & Victor's Principles Of Neurology** by Maurice Victor, et al; Hardcover - 1692 pages; 7th edition (December 19, 2000), McGraw-Hill Professional Publishing; ISBN: 0070674973; **http://www.amazon.com/exec/obidos/ASIN/0070674973/icongroupinterna**
- **American Academy of Pediatrics Guide to Your Child's Symptoms : The Official, Complete Home Reference, Birth Through Adolescence** by Donald Schiff (Editor), et al; Paperback - 256 pages (January 1997), Villard Books; ISBN: 0375752579; **http://www.amazon.com/exec/obidos/ASIN/0375752579/icongroupinterna**
- **The Children's Hospital Guide to Your Child's Health and Development** by Alan D. Woolf (Editor), et al; Hardcover - 796 pages, 1st edition (January 15, 2001), Perseus Books; ISBN: 073820241X; **http://www.amazon.com/exec/obidos/ASIN/073820241X/icongroupinterna**
- **Clinical Neuroanatomy Made Ridiculously Simple (MedMaster Series, 2000 Edition)** by Stephen Goldberg; Paperback: 97 pages; 2nd edition (February 15, 2000), Medmaster; ISBN: 0940780461; **http://www.amazon.com/exec/obidos/ASIN/0940780461/icongroupinterna**
- **Helping Your Child in the Hospital: A Practical Guide for Parents** by Nancy Keene, Rachel Prentice; Paperback - 176 pages, 3rd edition (April 15, 2002), O'Reilly & Associates; ISBN: 0596500114; **http://www.amazon.com/exec/obidos/ASIN/0596500114/icongroupinterna**
- **It's Not a Tumor!: The Patient's Guide to Common Neurological Problems** by Robert Wiedemeyer; Paperback: (January 1996), Boxweed Pub; ISBN: 0964740796; **http://www.amazon.com/exec/obidos/ASIN/0964740796/icongroupinterna**
- **Medical Emergencies & Childhood Illnesses: Includes Your Child's Personal Health Journal (Parent Smart)** by Penny A. Shore, William Sears (Contributor); Paperback - 115 pages (February 2002), Parent Kit Corporation; ISBN: 1896833187; **http://www.amazon.com/exec/obidos/ASIN/1896833187/icongroupinterna**

- **Neurology for the Non-Neurologist** by William J. Weiner (Editor), Christopher G. Goetz (Editor); Paperback (May 1999), Lippincott, Williams & Wilkins Publishers; ISBN: 0781717078; **http://www.amazon.com/exec/obidos/ASIN/0781717078/icongroupinterna**
- **Taking Care of Your Child: A Parent's Guide to Complete Medical Care** by Robert H. Pantell, M.D., et al; Paperback - 524 pages, 6th edition (March 5, 2002), Perseus Press; ISBN: 0738206016; **http://www.amazon.com/exec/obidos/ASIN/0738206016/icongroupinterna**

Vocabulary Builder

Arteriovenous: Both arterial and venous; pertaining to or affecting an artery and a vein. [EU]

Atrophy: A wasting away; a diminution in the size of a cell, tissue, organ, or part. [EU]

Cerebellar: Pertaining to the cerebellum. [EU]

Cerebrovascular: Pertaining to the blood vessels of the cerebrum, or brain. [EU]

Contusion: A bruise; an injury of a part without a break in the skin. [EU]

Dysplasia: Abnormality of development; in pathology, alteration in size, shape, and organization of adult cells. [EU]

Ganglioglioma: Rare indolent tumors comprised of neoplastic glial and neuronal cells which occur primarily in children and young adults. Benign lesions tend to be associated with long survival unless the tumor degenerates into a histologically malignant form. They tend to occur in the optic nerve and white matter of the brain and spinal cord. [NIH]

Hamartoma: A focal malformation resembling a neoplasm, composed of an overgrowth of mature cells and tissues that normally occur in the affected area. [NIH]

Hematoma: An extravasation of blood localized in an organ, space, or tissue. [NIH]

Hemorrhage: Bleeding or escape of blood from a vessel. [NIH]

Laceration: 1. The act of tearing. 2. A torn, ragged, mangled wound. [EU]

Neuroanatomy: Study of the anatomy of the nervous system as a specialty or discipline. [NIH]

Pediatrics: A medical specialty concerned with maintaining health and providing medical care to children from birth to adolescence. [NIH]

Vasculitis: Inflammation of a vessel, angiitis. [EU]

PART III. APPENDICES

ABOUT PART III

Part III is a collection of appendices on general medical topics relating to megalencephaly and related conditions.

Appendix A. Researching Your Child's Medications

Overview

There are a number of sources available on new or existing medications which could be prescribed to treat megalencephaly. While a number of hard copy or CD-Rom resources are available to parents and physicians for research purposes, a more flexible method is to use Internet-based databases. In this chapter, we will begin with a general overview of medications. We will then proceed to outline official recommendations on how you should view your child's medications. You may also want to research medications that your child is currently taking for other conditions as they may interact with medications for megalencephaly. Research can give you information on the side effects, interactions, and limitations of prescription drugs used in the treatment of megalencephaly. Broadly speaking, there are two sources of information on approved medications: public sources and private sources. We will emphasize free-to-use public sources.

Your Child's Medications: The Basics[17]

The Agency for Health Care Research and Quality has published extremely useful guidelines on the medication aspects of megalencephaly. Giving your child medication can involve many steps and decisions each day. The AHCRQ recommends that parents take part in treatment decisions. Do not be afraid to ask questions and talk about your concerns. By taking a moment to ask questions, your child may be spared from possible problems. Here are some points to cover each time a new medicine is prescribed:

---

[17] This section is adapted from AHCRQ: **http://www.ahcpr.gov/consumer/ncpiebro.htm** .

- Ask about all parts of your child's treatment, including diet changes, exercise, and medicines.
- Ask about the risks and benefits of each medicine or other treatment your child might receive.
- Ask how often you or your child's doctor will check for side effects from a given medication.

Do not hesitate to tell the doctor about preferences you have for your child's medicines. You may want your child to have a medicine with the fewest side effects, or the fewest doses to take each day. You may care most about cost. Or, you may want the medicine the doctor believes will work the best. Sharing your concerns will help the doctor select the best treatment for your child.

Do not be afraid to "bother" the doctor with your questions about medications for megalencephaly. You can also talk to a nurse or a pharmacist. They can help you better understand your child's treatment plan. Talking over your child's options with someone you trust can help you make better choices. Specifically, ask the doctor the following:

- The name of the medicine and what it is supposed to do.
- How and when to give your child the medicine, how much, and for how long.
- What food, drinks, other medicines, or activities your child should avoid while taking the medicine.
- What side effects your child may experience, and what to do if they occur.
- If there are any refills, and how often.
- About any terms or directions you do not understand.
- What to do if your child misses a dose.
- If there is written information you can take home (most pharmacies have information sheets on prescription medicines; some even offer large-print or Spanish versions).

Do not forget to tell the doctor about all the medicines your child is currently taking (not just those for megalencephaly). This includes prescription medicines and the medicines that you buy over the counter. When talking to the doctor, you may wish to prepare a list of medicines your child is currently taking including why and in what forms. Be sure to include the following information for each:

- Name of medicine
- Reason taken
- Dosage
- Time(s) of day

Also include any over-the-counter medicines, such as:

- Laxatives
- Diet pills
- Vitamins
- Cold medicine
- Aspirin or other pain, headache, or fever medicine
- Cough medicine
- Allergy relief medicine
- Antacids
- Sleeping pills
- Others (include names)

Learning More about Your Child's Medications

Because of historical investments by various organizations and the emergence of the Internet, it has become rather simple to learn about the medications the doctor has recommended for megalencephaly. One such source is the United States Pharmacopeia. In 1820, eleven physicians met in Washington, D.C. to establish the first compendium of standard drugs for the United States. They called this compendium the "U.S. Pharmacopeia (USP)." Today, the USP is a non-profit organization consisting of 800 volunteer scientists, eleven elected officials, and 400 representatives of state associations and colleges of medicine and pharmacy. The USP is located in Rockville, Maryland, and its home page is located at **www.usp.org**. The USP currently provides standards for over 3,700 medications. The resulting USP DI® Advice for the Patient® can be accessed through the National Library of

Medicine of the National Institutes of Health. The database is partially derived from lists of federally approved medications in the Food and Drug Administration's (FDA) Drug Approvals database.[18]

While the FDA database is rather large and difficult to navigate, the Phamacopeia is both user-friendly and free to use. It covers more than 9,000 prescription and over-the-counter medications. To access this database, simply type the following hyperlink into your Web browser: **http://www.nlm.nih.gov/medlineplus/druginformation.html**. To view examples of a given medication (brand names, category, description, preparation, proper use, precautions, side effects, etc.), simply follow the hyperlinks indicated within the United States Pharmacopeia (USP).

Commercial Databases

In addition to the medications listed in the USP above, a number of commercial sites are available by subscription to physicians and their institutions. You may be able to access these sources from your local medical library or your child's doctor's office.

Mosby's GenRx

Mosby's GenRx database (also available on CD-Rom and book format) covers 45,000 drug products including generics and international brands. It provides information on prescribing and drug interactions. Information can be obtained at the following hyperlink: **http://www.genrx.com/Mosby/PhyGenRx/group.html**.

PDR*health*

The PDR*health* database is a free-to-use, drug information search engine that has been written for the public in layman's terms. It contains FDA-approved drug information adapted from the Physicians' Desk Reference (PDR) database. PDR*health* can be searched by brand name, generic name, or indication. It features multiple drug interactions reports. Search PDR*health* at **http://www.pdrhealth.com/drug_info/index.html**.

[18] Though cumbersome, the FDA database can be freely browsed at the following site: **www.fda.gov/cder/da/da.htm**.

Other Web Sites

A number of additional Web sites discuss drug information. As an example, you may like to look at **www.drugs.com** which reproduces the information in the Pharmacopeia as well as commercial information. You may also want to consider the Web site of the Medical Letter, Inc. which allows users to download articles on various drugs and therapeutics for a nominal fee: **http://www.medletter.com/**.

Contraindications and Interactions (Hidden Dangers)

Some of the medications mentioned in the previous discussions can be problematic for children with megalencephaly--not because they are used in the treatment process, but because of contraindications, or side effects. Medications with contraindications are those that could react with drugs used to treat megalencephaly or potentially create deleterious side effects in patients with megalencephaly. You should ask the physician about any contraindications, especially as these might apply to other medications that your child may be taking for common ailments.

Drug-drug interactions occur when two or more drugs react with each other. This drug-drug interaction may cause your child to experience an unexpected side effect. Drug interactions may make medications less effective, cause unexpected side effects, or increase the action of a particular drug. Some drug interactions can even be harmful to your child.

Be sure to read the label every time you give your child a nonprescription or prescription drug, and take the time to learn about drug interactions. These precautions may be critical to your child's health. You can reduce the risk of potentially harmful drug interactions and side effects with a little bit of knowledge and common sense.

Drug labels contain important information about ingredients, uses, warnings, and directions which you should take the time to read and understand. Labels also include warnings about possible drug interactions. Further, drug labels may change as new information becomes avaiable. This is why it's especially important to read the label every time you give your child a medication. When the doctor prescribes a new drug, discuss all over-the-counter and prescription medications, dietary supplements, vitamins, botanicals, minerals and herbals your child takes. Ask your pharmacist for the package insert for each drug prescribed. The package insert provides more information about potential drug interactions.

A Final Warning

At some point, you may hear of alternative medications from friends, relatives, or in the news media. Advertisements may suggest that certain alternative drugs can produce positive results for megalencephaly. Exercise caution--some of these drugs may have fraudulent claims, and others may actually hurt your child. The Food and Drug Administration (FDA) is the official U.S. agency charged with discovering which medications are likely to improve the health of patients with megalencephaly. The FDA warns to watch out for[19]:

- Secret formulas (real scientists share what they know)
- Amazing breakthroughs or miracle cures (real breakthroughs don't happen very often; when they do, real scientists do not call them amazing or miracles)
- Quick, painless, or guaranteed cures
- If it sounds too good to be true, it probably isn't true.

If you have any questions about any kind of medical treatment, the FDA may have an office near you. Look for their number in the blue pages of the phone book. You can also contact the FDA through its toll-free number, 1-888-INFO-FDA (1-888-463-6332), or on the World Wide Web at **www.fda.gov**.

General References

In addition to the resources provided earlier in this chapter, the following general references describe medications (sorted alphabetically by title; hyperlinks provide rankings, information and reviews at Amazon.com):

- **Current Therapy in Neurologic Disease** by Richard T. Johnson, et al; Hardcover - 457 pages, 6th edition (January 15, 2002), Mosby-Year Book; ISBN: 0323014720; **http://www.amazon.com/exec/obidos/ASIN/0323014720/icongroupinterna**
- **Emerging Pharmacological Tools in Clinical Neurology** by MedPanel Inc. (Author); Digital - 66 pages, MarketResearch.com; ISBN: B00005RBN8;

[19] This section has been adapted from **http://www.fda.gov/opacom/lowlit/medfraud.html**

http://www.amazon.com/exec/obidos/ASIN/B00005RBN8/icongroupinterna

- **Goodman & Gilman's The Pharmacological Basis of Therapeutics by** Joel G. Hardman (Editor), Lee E. Limbird; Hardcover - 1825 pages, 10th edition (August 13, 2001), McGraw-Hill Professional Publishing; ISBN: 0071354697; **http://www.amazon.com/exec/obidos/ASIN/0071354697/icongroupinterna**
- **Neurology and General Medicine** by Michael J. Aminoff (Editor), Hardcover - 992 pages, 3rd edition (March 15, 2001), Churchill Livingstone; ISBN: 0443065713; **http://www.amazon.com/exec/obidos/ASIN/0443065713/icongroupinterna**
- **Neurology and Medicine** by Hughes Perkins; Hardcover - 415 pages, 1st edition (December 15, 1999), B. M. J. Books; ISBN: 0727912240; **http://www.amazon.com/exec/obidos/ASIN/0727912240/icongroupinterna**
- **Pharmacological Management of Neurological and Psychiatric Disorders** by S. J. Enna (Editor), et al; Hardcover - 736 pages, 1st edition, McGraw-Hill Professional Publishing; ISBN: 0070217645; **http://www.amazon.com/exec/obidos/ASIN/0070217645/icongroupinterna**

APPENDIX B. RESEARCHING NUTRITION

Overview

Since the time of Hippocrates, doctors have understood the importance of diet and nutrition to health and well-being. Since then, they have accumulated an impressive archive of studies and knowledge dedicated to this subject. Based on their experience, doctors and healthcare providers may recommend particular dietary supplements for megalencephaly. Any dietary recommendation is based on age, body mass, gender, lifestyle, eating habits, food preferences, and health condition. It is therefore likely that different patients with megalencephaly may be given different recommendations. Some recommendations may be directly related to megalencephaly, while others may be more related to general health.

In this chapter we will begin by briefly reviewing the essentials of diet and nutrition that will broadly frame more detailed discussions of megalencephaly. We will then show you how to find studies dedicated specifically to nutrition and megalencephaly.

Food and Nutrition: General Principles

What Are Essential Foods?

Food is generally viewed by official sources as consisting of six basic elements: (1) fluids, (2) carbohydrates, (3) protein, (4) fats, (5) vitamins, and (6) minerals. Consuming a combination of these elements is considered to be a healthy diet:

- **Fluids** are essential to human life as 80-percent of the body is composed of water. Water is lost via urination, sweating, diarrhea, vomiting, diuretics (drugs that increase urination), caffeine, and physical exertion.
- **Carbohydrates** are the main source for human energy (thermoregulation) and the bulk of typical diets. They are mostly classified as being either simple or complex. Simple carbohydrates include sugars which are often consumed in the form of cookies, candies, or cakes. Complex carbohydrates consist of starches and dietary fibers. Starches are consumed in the form of pastas, breads, potatoes, rice, and other foods. Soluble fibers can be eaten in the form of certain vegetables, fruits, oats, and legumes. Insoluble fibers include brown rice, whole grains, certain fruits, wheat bran and legumes.
- **Proteins** are eaten to build and repair human tissues. Some foods that are high in protein are also high in fat and calories. Food sources for protein include nuts, meat, fish, cheese, and other dairy products.
- **Fats** are consumed for both energy and the absorption of certain vitamins. There are many types of fats, with many general publications recommending the intake of unsaturated fats or those low in cholesterol.

Vitamins and minerals are fundamental to human health, growth, and, in some cases, disease prevention. Most are consumed in your child's diet (exceptions being vitamins K and D which are produced by intestinal bacteria and sunlight on the skin, respectively). Each vitamin and mineral plays a different role in health. The following outlines essential vitamins:

- **Vitamin A** is important to the health of eyes, hair, bones, and skin; sources of vitamin A include foods such as eggs, carrots, and cantaloupe.
- **Vitamin B^1**, also known as thiamine, is important for the nervous system and energy production; food sources for thiamine include meat, peas, fortified cereals, bread, and whole grains.
- **Vitamin B^2**, also known as riboflavin, is important for the nervous system and muscles, but is also involved in the release of proteins from nutrients; food sources for riboflavin include dairy products, leafy vegetables, meat, and eggs.
- **Vitamin B^3**, also known as niacin, is important for healthy skin and helps the body use energy; food sources for niacin include peas, peanuts, fish, and whole grains
- **Vitamin B^6**, also known as pyridoxine, is important for the regulation of cells in the nervous system and is vital for blood formation; food sources for pyridoxine include bananas, whole grains, meat, and fish.

- **Vitamin B^{12}** is vital for a healthy nervous system and for the growth of red blood cells in bone marrow; food sources for vitamin B^{12} include yeast, milk, fish, eggs, and meat.
- **Vitamin C** allows the body's immune system to fight various medical conditions, strengthens body tissue, and improves the body's use of iron; food sources for vitamin C include a wide variety of fruits and vegetables.
- **Vitamin D** helps the body absorb calcium which strengthens bones and teeth; food sources for vitamin D include oily fish and dairy products.
- **Vitamin E** can help protect certain organs and tissues from various degenerative diseases; food sources for vitamin E include margarine, vegetables, eggs, and fish.
- **Vitamin K** is essential for bone formation and blood clotting; common food sources for vitamin K include leafy green vegetables.
- **Folic Acid** maintains healthy cells and blood; food sources for folic acid include nuts, fortified breads, leafy green vegetables, and whole grains.

It should be noted that one can overdose on certain vitamins which become toxic if consumed in excess (e.g. vitamin A, D, E and K).

Like vitamins, minerals are chemicals that are required by the body to remain in good health. Because the human body does not manufacture these chemicals internally, we obtain them from food and other dietary sources. The more important minerals include:

- **Calcium** is needed for healthy bones, teeth, and muscles, but also helps the nervous system function; food sources for calcium include dry beans, peas, eggs, and dairy products.
- **Chromium** is helpful in regulating sugar levels in blood; food sources for chromium include egg yolks, raw sugar, cheese, nuts, beets, whole grains, and meat.
- **Fluoride** is used by the body to help prevent tooth decay and to reinforce bone strength; sources of fluoride include drinking water and certain brands of toothpaste.
- **Iodine** helps regulate the body's use of energy by synthesizing into the hormone thyroxine; food sources include leafy green vegetables, nuts, egg yolks, and red meat.
- **Iron** helps maintain muscles and the formation of red blood cells and certain proteins; food sources for iron include meat, dairy products, eggs, and leafy green vegetables.

- **Magnesium** is important for the production of DNA, as well as for healthy teeth, bones, muscles, and nerves; food sources for magnesium include dried fruit, dark green vegetables, nuts, and seafood.
- **Phosphorous** is used by the body to work with calcium to form bones and teeth; food sources for phosphorous include eggs, meat, cereals, and dairy products.
- **Selenium** primarily helps maintain normal heart and liver functions; food sources for selenium include wholegrain cereals, fish, meat, and dairy products.
- **Zinc** helps wounds heal, the formation of sperm, and encourage rapid growth and energy; food sources include dried beans, shellfish, eggs, and nuts.

The United States government periodically publishes recommended diets and consumption levels of the various elements of food. Again, the doctor may encourage deviations from the average official recommendation based on your child's specific condition. To learn more about basic dietary guidelines, visit the Web site: **http://www.health.gov/dietaryguidelines/**. Based on these guidelines, many foods are required to list the nutrition levels on the food's packaging. Labeling Requirements are listed at the following site maintained by the Food and Drug Administration: **http://www.cfsan.fda.gov/~dms/lab-cons.html**. When interpreting these requirements, the government recommends that consumers become familiar with the following abbreviations before reading FDA literature:[20]

- **DVs (Daily Values):** A new dietary reference term that will appear on the food label. It is made up of two sets of references, DRVs and RDIs.
- **DRVs (Daily Reference Values):** A set of dietary references that applies to fat, saturated fat, cholesterol, carbohydrate, protein, fiber, sodium, and potassium.
- **RDIs (Reference Daily Intakes):** A set of dietary references based on the Recommended Dietary Allowances for essential vitamins and minerals and, in selected groups, protein. The name "RDI" replaces the term "U.S. RDA."
- **RDAs (Recommended Dietary Allowances):** A set of estimated nutrient allowances established by the National Academy of Sciences. It is updated periodically to reflect current scientific knowledge.

[20] Adapted from the FDA: **http://www.fda.gov/fdac/special/foodlabel/dvs.html**.

What Are Dietary Supplements?[21]

Dietary supplements are widely available through many commercial sources, including health food stores, grocery stores, pharmacies, and by mail. Dietary supplements are provided in many forms including tablets, capsules, powders, gel-tabs, extracts, and liquids. Historically in the United States, the most prevalent type of dietary supplement was a multivitamin/mineral tablet or capsule that was available in pharmacies, either by prescription or "over the counter." Supplements containing strictly herbal preparations were less widely available. Currently in the United States, a wide array of supplement products are available, including vitamin, mineral, other nutrients, and botanical supplements as well as ingredients and extracts of animal and plant origin.

The Office of Dietary Supplements (ODS) of the National Institutes of Health is the official agency of the United States which has the expressed goal of acquiring "new knowledge to help prevent, detect, diagnose, and treat disease and disability, from the rarest genetic disorder to the common cold."[22] According to the ODS, dietary supplements can have an important impact on the prevention and management of medical conditions and on the maintenance of health.[23] The ODS notes that considerable research on the effects of dietary supplements has been conducted in Asia and Europe where the use of plant products, in particular, has a long tradition. However, the overwhelming majority of supplements have not been studied scientifically. To explore the role of dietary supplements in the improvement of health care, the ODS plans, organizes, and supports conferences, workshops, and symposia on scientific topics related to dietary supplements. The ODS often works in conjunction with other NIH Institutes and Centers, other government agencies, professional organizations, and public advocacy groups.

---

[21] This discussion has been adapted from the NIH:
http://ods.od.nih.gov/showpage.aspx?pageid=46.

[22] Contact: The Office of Dietary Supplements, National Institutes of Health, Building 31, Room 1B29, 31 Center Drive, MSC 2086, Bethesda, Maryland 20892-2086, Tel: (301) 435-2920, Fax: (301) 480-1845, E-mail: ods@nih.gov.

[23] Adapted from **http://ods.od.nih.gov/showpage.aspx?pageid=2**. The Dietary Supplement Health and Education Act defines dietary supplements as "a product (other than tobacco) intended to supplement the diet that bears or contains one or more of the following dietary ingredients: a vitamin, mineral, amino acid, herb or other botanical; or a dietary substance for use to supplement the diet by increasing the total detary intake; or a concentrate, metabolite, constituent, extract, or combination of any ingredient described above; and intended for ingestion in the form of a capsule, powder, softgel, or gelcap, and not represented as a conventional food or as a sole item of a meal or the diet."

To learn more about official information on dietary supplements, visit the ODS site at **http://ods.od.nih.gov/whatare/whatare.html**. Or contact:

The Office of Dietary Supplements
National Institutes of Health
Building 31, Room 1B29
31 Center Drive, MSC 2086
Bethesda, Maryland 20892-2086
Tel: (301) 435-2920
Fax: (301) 480-1845
E-mail: ods@nih.gov

Finding Studies on Megalencephaly

The NIH maintains an office dedicated to nutrition and diet. The National Institutes of Health's Office of Dietary Supplements (ODS) offers a searchable bibliographic database called the IBIDS (International Bibliographic Information on Dietary Supplements). The IBIDS contains over 460,000 scientific citations and summaries about dietary supplements and nutrition as well as references to published international, scientific literature on dietary supplements such as vitamins, minerals, and botanicals.[24] IBIDS is available to the public free of charge through the ODS Internet page: **http://ods.od.nih.gov/databases/ibids.html**.

After entering the search area, you have three choices: (1) IBIDS Consumer Database, (2) Full IBIDS Database, or (3) Peer Reviewed Citations Only. We recommend that you start with the Consumer Database. While you may not find references for the topics that are of most interest to you, check back periodically as this database is frequently updated. More studies can be found by searching the Full IBIDS Database. Healthcare professionals and researchers generally use the third option, which lists peer-reviewed citations. In all cases, we suggest that you take advantage of the "Advanced Search" option that allows you to retrieve up to 100 fully explained references in a comprehensive format. Type "megalencephaly" (or synonyms) into the search box. To narrow the search, you can also select the "Title" field.

---

24 Adapted from **http://ods.od.nih.gov**. IBIDS is produced by the Office of Dietary Supplements (ODS) at the National Institutes of Health to assist the public, healthcare providers, educators, and researchers in locating credible, scientific information on dietary supplements. IBIDS was developed and will be maintained through an interagency partnership with the Food and Nutrition Information Center of the National Agricultural Library, U.S. Department of Agriculture.

The following information is typical of that found when using the "Full IBIDS Database" when searching using "megalencephaly" (or a synonym):

- **Megalencephaly in the neonatal period as the initial manifestation of glutaric aciduria type I.**
  Author(s): Department of Pediatrics, Duke University Medical Center, Durham, North Carolina 27710.
  Source: Iafolla, A K Kahler, S G J-Pediatr. 1989 June; 114(6): 1004-6 0022-3476

Federal Resources on Nutrition

In addition to the IBIDS, the United States Department of Health and Human Services (HHS) and the United States Department of Agriculture (USDA) provide many sources of information on general nutrition and health. Recommended resources include:

- healthfinder®, HHS's gateway to health information, including diet and nutrition:
  http://www.healthfinder.gov/scripts/SearchContext.asp?topic=238&page=0
- The United States Department of Agriculture's Web site dedicated to nutrition information: **www.nutrition.gov**
- The Food and Drug Administration's Web site for federal food safety information: **www.foodsafety.gov**
- The National Action Plan on Overweight and Obesity sponsored by the United States Surgeon General:
  http://www.surgeongeneral.gov/topics/obesity/
- The Center for Food Safety and Applied Nutrition has an Internet site sponsored by the Food and Drug Administration and the Department of Health and Human Services: **http://vm.cfsan.fda.gov/**
- Center for Nutrition Policy and Promotion sponsored by the United States Department of Agriculture: **http://www.usda.gov/cnpp/**
- Food and Nutrition Information Center, National Agricultural Library sponsored by the United States Department of Agriculture: **http://www.nal.usda.gov/fnic/**
- Food and Nutrition Service sponsored by the United States Department of Agriculture: **http://www.fns.usda.gov/fns/**

Additional Web Resources

A number of additional Web sites offer encyclopedic information covering food and nutrition. The following is a representative sample:

- AOL: **http://search.aol.com/cat.adp?id=174&layer=&from=subcats**
- Family Village: **http://www.familyvillage.wisc.edu/med_nutrition.html**
- Google: **http://directory.google.com/Top/Health/Nutrition/**
- Open Directory Project: **http://dmoz.org/Health/Nutrition/**
- Yahoo.com: **http://dir.yahoo.com/Health/Nutrition/**
- WebMD®Health: **http://my.webmd.com/nutrition**
- WholeHealthMD.com: **http://www.wholehealthmd.com/reflib/0,1529,,00.html**

APPENDIX C. FINDING MEDICAL LIBRARIES

Overview

At a medical library you can find medical texts and reference books, consumer health publications, specialty newspapers and magazines, as well as medical journals. In this Appendix, we show you how to quickly find a medical library in your area.

Preparation

Before going to the library, highlight the references mentioned in this sourcebook that you find interesting. Focus on those items that are not available via the Internet, and ask the reference librarian for help with your search. He or she may know of additional resources that could be helpful to you. Most importantly, your local public library and medical libraries have Interlibrary Loan programs with the National Library of Medicine (NLM), one of the largest medical collections in the world. According to the NLM, most of the literature in the general and historical collections of the National Library of Medicine is available on interlibrary loan to any library. NLM's interlibrary loan services are only available to libraries. If you would like to access NLM medical literature, then visit a library in your area that can request the publications for you.[25]

[25] Adapted from the NLM: **http://www.nlm.nih.gov/psd/cas/interlibrary.html**

Finding a Local Medical Library

The quickest method to locate medical libraries is to use the Internet-based directory published by the National Network of Libraries of Medicine (NN/LM). This network includes 4626 members and affiliates that provide many services to librarians, health professionals, and the public. To find a library in your area, simply visit **http://nnlm.gov/members/adv.html** or call 1-800-338-7657.

Medical Libraries in the U.S. and Canada

In addition to the NN/LM, the National Library of Medicine (NLM) lists a number of libraries with reference facilities that are open to the public. The following is the NLM's list and includes hyperlinks to each library's Web site. These Web pages can provide information on hours of operation and other restrictions. The list below is a small sample of libraries recommended by the National Library of Medicine (sorted alphabetically by name of the U.S. state or Canadian province where the library is located)[26]:

- **Alabama:** Health InfoNet of Jefferson County (Jefferson County Library Cooperative, Lister Hill Library of the Health Sciences), **http://www.uab.edu/infonet/**
- **Alabama:** Richard M. Scrushy Library (American Sports Medicine Institute)
- **Arizona:** Samaritan Regional Medical Center: The Learning Center (Samaritan Health System, Phoenix, Arizona), **http://www.samaritan.edu/library/bannerlibs.htm**
- **California:** Kris Kelly Health Information Center (St. Joseph Health System, Humboldt), **http://www.humboldt1.com/~kkhic/index.html**
- **California:** Community Health Library of Los Gatos, **http://www.healthlib.org/orgresources.html**
- **California:** Consumer Health Program and Services (CHIPS) (County of Los Angeles Public Library, Los Angeles County Harbor-UCLA Medical Center Library) - Carson, CA, **http://www.colapublib.org/services/chips.html**
- **California:** Gateway Health Library (Sutter Gould Medical Foundation)
- **California:** Health Library (Stanford University Medical Center), **http://www-med.stanford.edu/healthlibrary/**

[26] Abstracted from **http://www.nlm.nih.gov/medlineplus/libraries.html**

- **California:** Patient Education Resource Center - Health Information and Resources (University of California, San Francisco), **http://sfghdean.ucsf.edu/barnett/PERC/default.asp**
- **California:** Redwood Health Library (Petaluma Health Care District), **http://www.phcd.org/rdwdlib.html**
- **California:** Los Gatos PlaneTree Health Library, **http://planetreesanjose.org/**
- **California:** Sutter Resource Library (Sutter Hospitals Foundation, Sacramento), **http://suttermedicalcenter.org/library/**
- **California:** Health Sciences Libraries (University of California, Davis), **http://www.lib.ucdavis.edu/healthsci/**
- **California:** ValleyCare Health Library & Ryan Comer Cancer Resource Center (ValleyCare Health System, Pleasanton), **http://gaelnet.stmarys-ca.edu/other.libs/gbal/east/vchl.html**
- **California:** Washington Community Health Resource Library (Fremont), **http://www.healthlibrary.org/**
- **Colorado:** William V. Gervasini Memorial Library (Exempla Healthcare), **http://www.saintjosephdenver.org/yourhealth/libraries/**
- **Connecticut:** Hartford Hospital Health Science Libraries (Hartford Hospital), **http://www.harthosp.org/library/**
- **Connecticut:** Healthnet: Connecticut Consumer Health Information Center (University of Connecticut Health Center, Lyman Maynard Stowe Library), **http://library.uchc.edu/departm/hnet/**
- **Connecticut:** Waterbury Hospital Health Center Library (Waterbury Hospital, Waterbury), **http://www.waterburyhospital.com/library/consumer.shtml**
- **Delaware:** Consumer Health Library (Christiana Care Health System, Eugene du Pont Preventive Medicine & Rehabilitation Institute, Wilmington), **http://www.christianacare.org/health_guide/health_guide_pmri_health_info.cfm**
- **Delaware:** Lewis B. Flinn Library (Delaware Academy of Medicine, Wilmington), **http://www.delamed.org/chls.html**
- **Georgia:** Family Resource Library (Medical College of Georgia, Augusta), **http://cmc.mcg.edu/kids_families/fam_resources/fam_res_lib/frl.htm**
- **Georgia:** Health Resource Center (Medical Center of Central Georgia, Macon), **http://www.mccg.org/hrc/hrchome.asp**

- **Hawaii:** Hawaii Medical Library: Consumer Health Information Service (Hawaii Medical Library, Honolulu), **http://hml.org/CHIS/**
- **Idaho:** DeArmond Consumer Health Library (Kootenai Medical Center, Coeur d'Alene), **http://www.nicon.org/DeArmond/index.htm**
- **Illinois:** Health Learning Center of Northwestern Memorial Hospital (Chicago), **http://www.nmh.org/health_info/hlc.html**
- **Illinois:** Medical Library (OSF Saint Francis Medical Center, Peoria), **http://www.osfsaintfrancis.org/general/library/**
- **Kentucky:** Medical Library - Services for Patients, Families, Students & the Public (Central Baptist Hospital, Lexington), **http://www.centralbap.com/education/community/library.cfm**
- **Kentucky:** University of Kentucky - Health Information Library (Chandler Medical Center, Lexington), **http://www.mc.uky.edu/PatientEd/**
- **Louisiana:** Alton Ochsner Medical Foundation Library (Alton Ochsner Medical Foundation, New Orleans), **http://www.ochsner.org/library/**
- **Louisiana:** Louisiana State University Health Sciences Center Medical Library-Shreveport, **http://lib-sh.lsuhsc.edu/**
- **Maine:** Franklin Memorial Hospital Medical Library (Franklin Memorial Hospital, Farmington), **http://www.fchn.org/fmh/lib.htm**
- **Maine:** Gerrish-True Health Sciences Library (Central Maine Medical Center, Lewiston), **http://www.cmmc.org/library/library.html**
- **Maine:** Hadley Parrot Health Science Library (Eastern Maine Healthcare, Bangor), **http://www.emh.org/hll/hpl/guide.htm**
- **Maine:** Maine Medical Center Library (Maine Medical Center, Portland), **http://www.mmc.org/library/**
- **Maine:** Parkview Hospital (Brunswick), **http://www.parkviewhospital.org/**
- **Maine:** Southern Maine Medical Center Health Sciences Library (Southern Maine Medical Center, Biddeford), **http://www.smmc.org/services/service.php3?choice=10**
- **Maine:** Stephens Memorial Hospital's Health Information Library (Western Maine Health, Norway), **http://www.wmhcc.org/Library/**
- **Manitoba, Canada:** Consumer & Patient Health Information Service (University of Manitoba Libraries), **http://www.umanitoba.ca/libraries/units/health/reference/chis.html**

- **Manitoba, Canada:** J.W. Crane Memorial Library (Deer Lodge Centre, Winnipeg), **http://www.deerlodge.mb.ca/crane_library/about.asp**
- **Maryland:** Health Information Center at the Wheaton Regional Library (Montgomery County, Dept. of Public Libraries, Wheaton Regional Library), **http://www.mont.lib.md.us/healthinfo/hic.asp**
- **Massachusetts:** Baystate Medical Center Library (Baystate Health System), **http://www.baystatehealth.com/1024/**
- **Massachusetts:** Boston University Medical Center Alumni Medical Library (Boston University Medical Center), **http://med-libwww.bu.edu/library/lib.html**
- **Massachusetts:** Lowell General Hospital Health Sciences Library (Lowell General Hospital, Lowell), **http://www.lowellgeneral.org/library/HomePageLinks/WWW.htm**
- **Massachusetts:** Paul E. Woodard Health Sciences Library (New England Baptist Hospital, Boston), **http://www.nebh.org/health_lib.asp**
- **Massachusetts:** St. Luke's Hospital Health Sciences Library (St. Luke's Hospital, Southcoast Health System, New Bedford), **http://www.southcoast.org/library/**
- **Massachusetts:** Treadwell Library Consumer Health Reference Center (Massachusetts General Hospital), **http://www.mgh.harvard.edu/library/chrcindex.html**
- **Massachusetts:** UMass HealthNet (University of Massachusetts Medical School, Worchester), **http://healthnet.umassmed.edu/**
- **Michigan:** Botsford General Hospital Library - Consumer Health (Botsford General Hospital, Library & Internet Services), **http://www.botsfordlibrary.org/consumer.htm**
- **Michigan:** Helen DeRoy Medical Library (Providence Hospital and Medical Centers), **http://www.providence-hospital.org/library/**
- **Michigan:** Marquette General Hospital - Consumer Health Library (Marquette General Hospital, Health Information Center), **http://www.mgh.org/center.html**
- **Michigan:** Patient Education Resouce Center - University of Michigan Cancer Center (University of Michigan Comprehensive Cancer Center, Ann Arbor), **http://www.cancer.med.umich.edu/learn/leares.htm**
- **Michigan:** Sladen Library & Center for Health Information Resources - Consumer Health Information (Detroit), **http://www.henryford.com/body.cfm?id=39330**

- **Montana:** Center for Health Information (St. Patrick Hospital and Health Sciences Center, Missoula)
- **National:** Consumer Health Library Directory (Medical Library Association, Consumer and Patient Health Information Section), **http://caphis.mlanet.org/directory/index.html**
- **National:** National Network of Libraries of Medicine (National Library of Medicine) - provides library services for health professionals in the United States who do not have access to a medical library, **http://nnlm.gov/**
- **National:** NN/LM List of Libraries Serving the Public (National Network of Libraries of Medicine), **http://nnlm.gov/members/**
- **Nevada:** Health Science Library, West Charleston Library (Las Vegas-Clark County Library District, Las Vegas), **http://www.lvccld.org/special_collections/medical/index.htm**
- **New Hampshire:** Dartmouth Biomedical Libraries (Dartmouth College Library, Hanover), **http://www.dartmouth.edu/~biomed/resources.htmld/conshealth.htmld**
- **New Jersey:** Consumer Health Library (Rahway Hospital, Rahway), **http://www.rahwayhospital.com/library.htm**
- **New Jersey:** Dr. Walter Phillips Health Sciences Library (Englewood Hospital and Medical Center, Englewood), **http://www.englewoodhospital.com/links/index.htm**
- **New Jersey:** Meland Foundation (Englewood Hospital and Medical Center, Englewood), **http://www.geocities.com/ResearchTriangle/9360/**
- **New York:** Choices in Health Information (New York Public Library) - NLM Consumer Pilot Project participant, **http://www.nypl.org/branch/health/links.html**
- **New York:** Health Information Center (Upstate Medical University, State University of New York, Syracuse), **http://www.upstate.edu/library/hic/**
- **New York:** Health Sciences Library (Long Island Jewish Medical Center, New Hyde Park), **http://www.lij.edu/library/library.html**
- **New York:** ViaHealth Medical Library (Rochester General Hospital), **http://www.nyam.org/library/**
- **Ohio:** Consumer Health Library (Akron General Medical Center, Medical & Consumer Health Library), **http://www.akrongeneral.org/hwlibrary.htm**

- **Oklahoma:** The Health Information Center at Saint Francis Hospital (Saint Francis Health System, Tulsa), **http://www.sfh-tulsa.com/services/healthinfo.asp**
- **Oregon:** Planetree Health Resource Center (Mid-Columbia Medical Center, The Dalles), **http://www.mcmc.net/phrc/**
- **Pennsylvania:** Community Health Information Library (Milton S. Hershey Medical Center, Hershey), **http://www.hmc.psu.edu/commhealth/**
- **Pennsylvania:** Community Health Resource Library (Geisinger Medical Center, Danville), **http://www.geisinger.edu/education/commlib.shtml**
- **Pennsylvania:** HealthInfo Library (Moses Taylor Hospital, Scranton), **http://www.mth.org/healthwellness.html**
- **Pennsylvania:** Hopwood Library (University of Pittsburgh, Health Sciences Library System, Pittsburgh), **http://www.hsls.pitt.edu/guides/chi/hopwood/index_html**
- **Pennsylvania:** Koop Community Health Information Center (College of Physicians of Philadelphia), **http://www.collphyphil.org/kooppg1.shtml**
- **Pennsylvania:** Learning Resources Center - Medical Library (Susquehanna Health System, Williamsport), **http://www.shscares.org/services/lrc/index.asp**
- **Pennsylvania:** Medical Library (UPMC Health System, Pittsburgh), **http://www.upmc.edu/passavant/library.htm**
- **Quebec, Canada:** Medical Library (Montreal General Hospital), **http://www.mghlib.mcgill.ca/**
- **South Dakota:** Rapid City Regional Hospital Medical Library (Rapid City Regional Hospital), **http://www.rcrh.org/Services/Library/Default.asp**
- **Texas:** Houston HealthWays (Houston Academy of Medicine-Texas Medical Center Library), **http://hhw.library.tmc.edu/**
- **Washington:** Community Health Library (Kittitas Valley Community Hospital), **http://www.kvch.com/**
- **Washington:** Southwest Washington Medical Center Library (Southwest Washington Medical Center, Vancouver), **http://www.swmedicalcenter.com/body.cfm?id=72**

APPENDIX D. YOUR CHILD'S RIGHTS AND INSURANCE

Overview

Parents face a series of issues related more to the healthcare industry than to their children's medical conditions. This appendix covers two important topics in this regard: your responsibilities and your child's rights as a patient, and how to get the most out of your child's medical insurance plan.

Your Child's Rights as a Patient

The President's Advisory Commission on Consumer Protection and Quality in the Healthcare Industry has created the following summary of your child's rights as a patient.[27]

[27] Adapted from Consumer Bill of Rights and Responsibilities: **http://www.hcqualitycommission.gov/press/cbor.html#head1**.

Information Disclosure

Consumers have the right to receive accurate, easily understood information. Some consumers require assistance in making informed decisions about health plans, health professionals, and healthcare facilities. Such information includes:

- ***Health plans.*** Covered benefits, cost-sharing, and procedures for resolving complaints, licensure, certification, and accreditation status, comparable measures of quality and consumer satisfaction, provider network composition, the procedures that govern access to specialists and emergency services, and care management information.
- ***Health professionals.*** Education, board certification, and recertification, years of practice, experience performing certain procedures, and comparable measures of quality and consumer satisfaction.
- ***Healthcare facilities.*** Experience in performing certain procedures and services, accreditation status, comparable measures of quality, worker, and consumer satisfaction, and procedures for resolving complaints.
- ***Consumer assistance programs.*** Programs must be carefully structured to promote consumer confidence and to work cooperatively with health plans, providers, payers, and regulators. Desirable characteristics of such programs are sponsorship that ensures accountability to the interests of consumers and stable, adequate funding.

Choice of Providers and Plans

Consumers have the right to a choice of healthcare providers that is sufficient to ensure access to appropriate high-quality healthcare. To ensure such choice, the Commission recommends the following:

- ***Provider network adequacy.*** All health plan networks should provide access to sufficient numbers and types of providers to assure that all covered services will be accessible without unreasonable delay -- including access to emergency services 24 hours a day and 7 days a week. If a health plan has an insufficient number or type of providers to provide a covered benefit with the appropriate degree of specialization, the plan should ensure that the consumer obtains the benefit outside the network at no greater cost than if the benefit were obtained from participating providers.
- ***Access to specialists.*** Consumers with complex or serious medical conditions who require frequent specialty care should have direct access

to a qualified specialist of their choice within a plan's network of providers. Authorizations, when required, should be for an adequate number of direct access visits under an approved treatment plan.

- *Transitional care.* Consumers who are undergoing a course of treatment for a chronic or disabling condition at the time they involuntarily change health plans or at a time when a provider is terminated by a plan for other than cause should be able to continue seeing their current specialty providers for up to 90 days to allow for transition of care.
- *Choice of health plans.* Public and private group purchasers should, wherever feasible, offer consumers a choice of high-quality health insurance plans.

Access to Emergency Services

Consumers have the right to access emergency healthcare services when and where the need arises. Health plans should provide payment when a consumer presents to an emergency department with acute symptoms of sufficient severity--including severe pain--such that a "prudent layperson" could reasonably expect the absence of medical attention to result in placing that consumer's health in serious jeopardy, serious impairment to bodily functions, or serious dysfunction of any bodily organ or part.

Participation in Treatment Decisions

Consumers have the right and responsibility to fully participate in all decisions related to their healthcare. Consumers who are unable to fully participate in treatment decisions have the right to be represented by parents, guardians, family members, or other conservators. Physicians and other health professionals should:

- Provide parents with sufficient information and opportunity to decide among treatment options consistent with the informed consent process.
- Discuss all treatment options with a parent in a culturally competent manner, including the option of no treatment at all.
- Ensure that persons with disabilities have effective communications with members of the health system in making such decisions.
- Discuss all current treatments a consumer may be undergoing.
- Discuss all risks, benefits, and consequences to treatment or nontreatment.

- Give parents the opportunity to refuse treatment for their children and to express preferences about future treatment decisions.
- Discuss the use of advance directives -- both living wills and durable powers of attorney for healthcare -- with parents.
- Abide by the decisions made by parents consistent with the informed consent process.

Health plans, health providers, and healthcare facilities should:

- Disclose to consumers factors -- such as methods of compensation, ownership of or interest in healthcare facilities, or matters of conscience -- that could influence advice or treatment decisions.
- Assure that provider contracts do not contain any so-called "gag clauses" or other contractual mechanisms that restrict healthcare providers' ability to communicate with and advise parents about medically necessary treatment options for their children.
- Be prohibited from penalizing or seeking retribution against healthcare professionals or other health workers for advocating on behalf of their patients.

Respect and Nondiscrimination

Consumers have the right to considerate, respectful care from all members of the healthcare industry at all times and under all circumstances. An environment of mutual respect is essential to maintain a quality healthcare system. To assure that right, the Commission recommends the following:

- Consumers must not be discriminated against in the delivery of healthcare services consistent with the benefits covered in their policy, or as required by law, based on race, ethnicity, national origin, religion, sex, age, mental or physical disability, sexual orientation, genetic information, or source of payment.
- Consumers eligible for coverage under the terms and conditions of a health plan or program, or as required by law, must not be discriminated against in marketing and enrollment practices based on race, ethnicity, national origin, religion, sex, age, mental or physical disability, sexual orientation, genetic information, or source of payment.

Confidentiality of Health Information

Consumers have the right to communicate with healthcare providers in confidence and to have the confidentiality of their individually identifiable healthcare information protected. Consumers also have the right to review and copy their own medical records and request amendments to their records.

Complaints and Appeals

Consumers have the right to a fair and efficient process for resolving differences with their health plans, healthcare providers, and the institutions that serve them, including a rigorous system of internal review and an independent system of external review. A free copy of the Patient's Bill of Rights is available from the American Hospital Association.[28]

Parent Responsibilities

To underscore the importance of finance in modern healthcare as well as your responsibility for the financial aspects of your child's care, the President's Advisory Commission on Consumer Protection and Quality in the Healthcare Industry has proposed that parents understand the following "Consumer Responsibilities."[29] In a healthcare system that protects consumers' rights, it is reasonable to expect and encourage consumers to assume certain responsibilities. Greater involvement by parents in their children's care increases the likelihood of achieving the best outcome and helps support a quality-oriented, cost-conscious environment. Such responsibilities include:

- Take responsibility for maximizing your child's healthy habits.
- Work collaboratively with healthcare providers in developing and carrying out your child's agreed-upon treatment plans.
- Disclose relevant information and clearly communicate wants and needs.
- Use the insurance company's internal complaint and appeal processes to address your concerns.
- Recognize the reality of risks, the limits of the medical science, and the human fallibility of the healthcare professional.

---

[28] To order your free copy of the Patient's Bill of Rights, telephone 312-422-3000 or visit the American Hospital Association's Web site: **http://www.aha.org**. Click on "Resource Center," go to "Search" at bottom of page, and then type in "Patient's Bill of Rights." The Patient's Bill of Rights is also available from Fax on Demand, at 312-422-2020, document number 471124.

[29] Adapted from **http://www.hcqualitycommission.gov/press/cbor.html#head1**.

- Be aware of a healthcare provider's obligation to be reasonably efficient and equitable in providing care to the community.
- Become knowledgeable about health plan coverage and options (when available) including all covered benefits, limitations, and exclusions, rules regarding use of network providers, coverage and referral rules, appropriate processes to secure additional information, and the process to appeal coverage decisions.
- Make a good-faith effort to meet financial obligations.
- Abide by administrative and operational procedures of health plans, healthcare providers, and Government health benefit programs.

Choosing an Insurance Plan

There are a number of official government agencies that help consumers understand their healthcare insurance choices.[30] The U.S. Department of Labor, in particular, recommends ten ways to make your health benefits choices work best for your family.[31]

1. Your options are important. There are many different types of health benefit plans. Find out which one your employer offers, then check out the plan, or plans, offered. Your employer's human resource office, the health plan administrator, or your union can provide information to help you match your family's needs and preferences with the available plans. The more information you have, the better your healthcare decisions will be.

2. Reviewing the benefits available. Do the plans offered cover preventive care, well-baby care, vision or dental care? Are there deductibles? Answers to these questions can help determine the out-of-pocket expenses you may face. Cheapest may not always be best. Your goal is high quality health benefits.

3. Look for quality. The quality of healthcare services varies, but quality can be measured. You should consider the quality of healthcare in deciding among the healthcare plans or options available to your family. Not all health plans, doctors, hospitals and other providers give the highest quality care. Fortunately, there is quality information you can use right now to help you compare your healthcare choices. Find out how you can measure

[30] More information about quality across programs is provided at the following AHRQ Web site: **http://www.ahrq.gov/consumer/qntascii/qnthplan.htm**.

[31] Adapted from the Department of Labor: **http://www.dol.gov/dol/pwba/public/pubs/health/top10-text.html**.

quality. Consult the U.S. Department of Health and Human Services publication "Your Guide to Choosing Quality Health Care" on the Internet at **www.ahcpr.gov/consumer.**

4. Your plan's summary plan description (SPD) provides a wealth of information. Your health plan administrator can provide you with a copy of your plan's SPD. It outlines your family's benefits and your legal rights under the Employee Retirement Income Security Act (ERISA), the federal law that protects your family's health benefits. It should contain information about the coverage of dependents, what services will require a co-pay, and the circumstances under which your employer can change or terminate a health benefits plan. Save the SPD and all other health plan brochures and documents, along with memos or correspondence from your employer relating to health benefits.

5. Assess your benefit coverage as your family status changes. Marriage, divorce, childbirth or adoption, and the death of a spouse are all life events that may signal a need to change your health benefits. You, your spouse and dependent children may be eligible for a special enrollment period under provisions of the Health Insurance Portability and Accountability Act (HIPAA). Even without life-changing events, the information provided by your employer should tell you how you can change benefits or switch plans, if more than one plan is offered. If your spouse's employer also offers a health benefits package, consider coordinating both plans for maximum coverage.

6. Changing jobs and other life events can affect your family's health benefits. Under the Consolidated Omnibus Budget Reconciliation Act (COBRA), you, your covered spouse, and your dependent children may be eligible to purchase extended health coverage under your employer's plan if you lose your job, change employers, get divorced, or upon occurrence of certain other events. Coverage can range from 18 to 36 months depending on your situation. COBRA applies to most employers with 20 or more workers and requires your plan to notify you of your rights. Most plans require eligible individuals to make their COBRA election within 60 days of the plan's notice. Be sure to follow up with your plan sponsor if you don't receive notice, and make sure you respond within the allotted time.

7. HIPAA can also help if you are changing jobs, particularly if you have a medical condition. HIPAA generally limits pre-existing condition exclusions to a maximum of 12 months (18 months for late enrollees). HIPAA also requires this maximum period to be reduced by the length of time you had prior "creditable coverage." You should receive a certificate documenting your prior creditable coverage from your old plan when coverage ends.

8. Plan for retirement. Before you retire, find out what health benefits, if any, extend to you and your spouse during your retirement years. Consult with your employer's human resources office, your union, the plan administrator, and check your SPD. Make sure there is no conflicting information among these sources about the benefits your family will receive or the circumstances under which they can change or be eliminated. With this information in hand, you can make other important choices, like finding out if you are eligible for Medicare and Medigap insurance coverage.

9. Know how to file an appeal if a health benefits claim is denied. Understand how your plan handles grievances and where to make appeals of the plan's decisions. Keep records and copies of correspondence. Check your health benefits package and your SPD to determine who is responsible for handling problems with benefit claims. Contact PWBA for customer service assistance if you are unable to obtain a response to your complaint.

10. You can take steps to improve the quality of the healthcare and the health benefits your family receives. Look for and use things like Quality Reports and Accreditation Reports whenever you can. Quality reports may contain consumer ratings -- how satisfied consumers are with the doctors in their plan, for instance-- and clinical performance measures -- how well a healthcare organization prevents and treats illness. Accreditation reports provide information on how accredited organizations meet national standards, and often include clinical performance measures. Look for these quality measures whenever possible. Consult "Your Guide to Choosing Quality Health Care" on the Internet at **www.ahcpr.gov/consumer**.

Medicaid

Illness strikes both rich and poor families. For low-income families, Medicaid is available to defer the costs of treatment. In the following pages, you will learn the basics about Medicaid as well as useful contact information on how to find more in-depth information.

Medicaid is a joint federal and state program that helps pay medical costs for some people with low incomes and limited resources. Medicaid programs vary from state to state. You can find more information about Medicaid on the HCFA.gov Web site at **http://www.hcfa.gov/medicaid/medicaid.htm**.

NORD's Medication Assistance Programs

Finally, the National Organization for Rare Disorders, Inc. (NORD) administers medication programs sponsored by humanitarian-minded pharmaceutical and biotechnology companies to help uninsured or under-insured individuals secure life-saving or life-sustaining drugs.[32] NORD programs ensure that certain vital drugs are available "to those families whose income is too high to qualify for Medicaid but too low to pay for their prescribed medications." The program has standards for fairness, equity, and unbiased eligibility. It currently covers some 14 programs for nine pharmaceutical companies. NORD also offers early access programs for investigational new drugs (IND) under the approved "Treatment INDs" programs of the Food and Drug Administration (FDA). In these programs, a limited number of individuals can receive investigational drugs that have yet to be approved by the FDA. These programs are generally designed for rare medical conditions. For more information, visit **www.rarediseases.org**.

Additional Resources

In addition to the references already listed in this chapter, you may need more information on health insurance, hospitals, or the healthcare system in general. The NIH has set up an excellent guidance Web site that addresses these and other issues. Topics include:[33]

- Health Insurance: **http://www.nlm.nih.gov/medlineplus/healthinsurance.html**
- Health Statistics: **http://www.nlm.nih.gov/medlineplus/healthstatistics.html**
- HMO and Managed Care: **http://www.nlm.nih.gov/medlineplus/managedcare.html**
- Hospice Care: **http://www.nlm.nih.gov/medlineplus/hospicecare.html**
- Medicaid: **http://www.nlm.nih.gov/medlineplus/medicaid.html**
- Medicare: **http://www.nlm.nih.gov/medlineplus/medicare.html**
- Nursing Homes and Long-Term Care: **http://www.nlm.nih.gov/medlineplus/nursinghomes.html**

---

[32] Adapted from NORD: **http://www.rarediseases.org/programs/medication**.

[33] You can access this information at: **http://www.nlm.nih.gov/medlineplus/healthsystem.html**.

- Patient's Rights, Confidentiality, Informed Consent, Ombudsman Programs, Privacy and Patient Issues: **http://www.nlm.nih.gov/medlineplus/patientissues.html**
- Veteran's Health, Persian Gulf War, Gulf War Syndrome, Agent Orange: **http://www.nlm.nih.gov/medlineplus/veteranshealth.html**

Vocabulary Builder

Capsules: Hard or soft soluble containers used for the oral administration of medicine. [NIH]

Carbohydrate: An aldehyde or ketone derivative of a polyhydric alcohol, particularly of the pentahydric and hexahydric alcohols. They are so named because the hydrogen and oxygen are usually in the proportion to form water, (CH2O)n. The most important carbohydrates are the starches, sugars, celluloses, and gums. They are classified into mono-, di-, tri-, poly- and heterosaccharides. [EU]

Cholesterol: The principal sterol of all higher animals, distributed in body tissues, especially the brain and spinal cord, and in animal fats and oils. [NIH]

Diarrhea: Passage of excessively liquid or excessively frequent stools. [NIH]

Iodine: A nonmetallic element of the halogen group that is represented by the atomic symbol I, atomic number 53, and atomic weight of 126.90. It is a nutritionally essential element, especially important in thyroid hormone synthesis. In solution, it has anti-infective properties and is used topically. [NIH]

Neonatal: Pertaining to the first four weeks after birth. [EU]

Niacin: Water-soluble vitamin of the B complex occurring in various animal and plant tissues. Required by the body for the formation of coenzymes NAD and NADP. Has pellagra-curative, vasodilating, and antilipemic properties. [NIH]

Overdose: 1. to administer an excessive dose. 2. an excessive dose. [EU]

Potassium: An element that is in the alkali group of metals. It has an atomic symbol K, atomic number 19, and atomic weight 39.10. It is the chief cation in the intracellular fluid of muscle and other cells. Potassium ion is a strong electrolyte and it plays a significant role in the regulation of fluid volume and maintenance of the water-electrolyte balance. [NIH]

Proteins: Polymers of amino acids linked by peptide bonds. The specific sequence of amino acids determines the shape and function of the protein. [NIH]

Riboflavin: Nutritional factor found in milk, eggs, malted barley, liver, kidney, heart, and leafy vegetables. The richest natural source is yeast. It occurs in the free form only in the retina of the eye, in whey, and in urine; its principal forms in tissues and cells are as FMN and FAD. [NIH]

Selenium: An element with the atomic symbol Se, atomic number 34, and atomic weight 78.96. It is an essential micronutrient for mammals and other animals but is toxic in large amounts. Selenium protects intracellular structures against oxidative damage. It is an essential component of glutathione peroxidase. [NIH]

Thermoregulation: Heat regulation. [EU]

Thyroxine: An amino acid of the thyroid gland which exerts a stimulating effect on thyroid metabolism. [NIH]

Toxic: Pertaining to, due to, or of the nature of a poison or toxin; manifesting the symptoms of severe infection. [EU]

ONLINE GLOSSARIES

The Internet provides access to a number of free-to-use medical dictionaries and glossaries. The National Library of Medicine has compiled the following list of online dictionaries:

- ADAM Medical Encyclopedia (A.D.A.M., Inc.), comprehensive medical reference: **http://www.nlm.nih.gov/medlineplus/encyclopedia.html**
- MedicineNet.com Medical Dictionary (MedicineNet, Inc.): **http://www.medterms.com/Script/Main/hp.asp**
- Merriam-Webster Medical Dictionary (Inteli-Health, Inc.): **http://www.intelihealth.com/IH/**
- Multilingual Glossary of Technical and Popular Medical Terms in Eight European Languages (European Commission) - Danish, Dutch, English, French, German, Italian, Portuguese, and Spanish: **http://allserv.rug.ac.be/~rvdstich/eugloss/welcome.html**
- On-line Medical Dictionary (CancerWEB): **http://www.graylab.ac.uk/omd/**
- Technology Glossary (National Library of Medicine) - Health Care Technology: **http://www.nlm.nih.gov/nichsr/ta101/ta10108.htm**
- Terms and Definitions (Office of Rare Diseases): **http://rarediseases.info.nih.gov/ord/glossary_a-e.html**

Beyond these, MEDLINEplus contains a very user-friendly encyclopedia covering every aspect of medicine (licensed from A.D.A.M., Inc.). The ADAM Medical Encyclopedia can be accessed via the following Web site address: **http://www.nlm.nih.gov/medlineplus/encyclopedia.html**. ADAM is also available on commercial Web sites such as Web MD (**http://my.webmd.com/adam/asset/adam_disease_articles/a_to_z/a**) and drkoop.com (**http://www.drkoop.com/**). Topics of interest can be researched by using keywords before continuing elsewhere, as these basic definitions and concepts will be useful in more advanced areas of research. You may choose to print various pages specifically relating to megalencephaly and keep them on file.

Online Dictionary Directories

The following are additional online directories compiled by the National Library of Medicine, including a number of specialized medical dictionaries and glossaries:

- Medical Dictionaries: Medical & Biological (World Health Organization): **http://www.who.int/hlt/virtuallibrary/English/diction.htm#Medical**
- MEL-Michigan Electronic Library List of Online Health and Medical Dictionaries (Michigan Electronic Library): **http://mel.lib.mi.us/health/health-dictionaries.html**
- Patient Education: Glossaries (DMOZ Open Directory Project): **http://dmoz.org/Health/Education/Patient_Education/Glossaries/**
- Web of Online Dictionaries (Bucknell University): **http://www.yourdictionary.com/diction5.html#medicine**

MEGALENCEPHALY GLOSSARY

The following is a complete glossary of terms used in this sourcebook. The definitions are derived from official public sources including the National Institutes of Health [NIH] and the European Union [EU]. After this glossary, we list a number of additional hardbound and electronic glossaries and dictionaries that you may wish to consult.

Anticonvulsant: An agent that prevents or relieves convulsions. [EU]

Arteriovenous: Both arterial and venous; pertaining to or affecting an artery and a vein. [EU]

Atrophy: A wasting away; a diminution in the size of a cell, tissue, organ, or part. [EU]

Bilateral: Having two sides, or pertaining to both sides. [EU]

Capsules: Hard or soft soluble containers used for the oral administration of medicine. [NIH]

Carbohydrate: An aldehyde or ketone derivative of a polyhydric alcohol, particularly of the pentahydric and hexahydric alcohols. They are so named because the hydrogen and oxygen are usually in the proportion to form water, (CH2O)n. The most important carbohydrates are the starches, sugars, celluloses, and gums. They are classified into mono-, di-, tri-, poly- and heterosaccharides. [EU]

Cardiovascular: Pertaining to the heart and blood vessels. [EU]

Cerebellar: Pertaining to the cerebellum. [EU]

Cerebellum: Part of the metencephalon that lies in the posterior cranial fossa behind the brain stem. It is concerned with the coordination of movement. [NIH]

Cerebral: Of or pertaining of the cerebrum or the brain. [EU]

Cerebrospinal: Pertaining to the brain and spinal cord. [EU]

Cerebrovascular: Pertaining to the blood vessels of the cerebrum, or brain. [EU]

Cholesterol: The principal sterol of all higher animals, distributed in body tissues, especially the brain and spinal cord, and in animal fats and oils. [NIH]

Chromosomal: Pertaining to chromosomes. [EU]

Chronic: Persisting over a long period of time. [EU]

Consciousness: Sense of awareness of self and of the environment. [NIH]

Contracture: A condition of fixed high resistance to passive stretch of a muscle, resulting from fibrosis of the tissues supporting the muscles or the joints, or from disorders of the muscle fibres. [EU]

Contusion: A bruise; an injury of a part without a break in the skin. [EU]

Convulsion: A violent involuntary contraction or series of contractions of the voluntary muscles. [EU]

Cortex: The outer layer of an organ or other body structure, as distinguished from the internal substance. [EU]

Cortical: Pertaining to or of the nature of a cortex or bark. [EU]

Cranial: Pertaining to the cranium, or to the anterior (in animals) or superior (in humans) end of the body. [EU]

Cyst: Any closed cavity or sac; normal or abnormal, lined by epithelium, and especially one that contains a liquid or semisolid material. [EU]

Dentists: Individuals licensed to practice dentistry. [NIH]

Diarrhea: Passage of excessively liquid or excessively frequent stools. [NIH]

Dysplasia: Abnormality of development; in pathology, alteration in size, shape, and organization of adult cells. [EU]

Embryo: In animals, those derivatives of the fertilized ovum that eventually become the offspring, during their period of most rapid development, i.e., after the long axis appears until all major structures are represented. In man, the developing organism is an embryo from about two weeks after fertilization to the end of seventh or eighth week. [EU]

Facial: Of or pertaining to the face. [EU]

Ganglioglioma: Rare indolent tumors comprised of neoplastic glial and neuronal cells which occur primarily in children and young adults. Benign lesions tend to be associated with long survival unless the tumor degenerates into a histologically malignant form. They tend to occur in the optic nerve and white matter of the brain and spinal cord. [NIH]

Gastrointestinal: Pertaining to or communicating with the stomach and intestine, as a gastrointestinal fistula. [EU]

Gastrostomy: Creation of an artificial external opening into the stomach for nutritional support or gastrointestinal compression. [NIH]

Hamartoma: A focal malformation resembling a neoplasm, composed of an overgrowth of mature cells and tissues that normally occur in the affected area. [NIH]

Hematoma: An extravasation of blood localized in an organ, space, or tissue. [NIH]

Hemorrhage: Bleeding or escape of blood from a vessel. [NIH]

Hernia: (he protrusion of a loop or knuckle of an organ or tissue through an abnormal opening. [EU]

Hydrocephalus: A condition marked by dilatation of the cerebral ventricles, most often occurring secondarily to obstruction of the cerebrospinal fluid pathways, and accompanied by an accumulation of cerebrospinal fluid within the skull; the fluid is usually under increased pressure, but occasionally may be normal or nearly so. It is typically characterized by enlargement of the head, prominence of the forehead, brain atrophy, mental deterioration, and convulsions; may be congenital or acquired; and may be of sudden onset (acute h.) or be slowly progressive (chronic or primary b.). [EU]

Hypertonia: Or hypertony n, pl. hypertonias or hypertonies : hypertonicity. n. Pathology: increased rigidity, tension and spasticity of the muscles. [EU]

Hypotonia: A condition of diminished tone of the skeletal muscles; diminished resistance of muscles to passive stretching. [EU]

Idiopathic: Of the nature of an idiopathy; self-originated; of unknown causation. [EU]

Infantile: Pertaining to an infant or to infancy. [EU]

Iodine: A nonmetallic element of the halogen group that is represented by the atomic symbol I, atomic number 53, and atomic weight of 126.90. It is a nutritionally essential element, especially important in thyroid hormone synthesis. In solution, it has anti-infective properties and is used topically. [NIH]

Jews: An ethnic group with certain cultural and religious traditions. [NIH]

Laceration: 1. The act of tearing. 2. A torn, ragged, mangled wound. [EU]

Lesion: Any pathological or traumatic discontinuity of tissue or loss of function of a part. [EU]

Lethal: Deadly, fatal. [EU]

Lip: Either of the two fleshy, full-blooded margins of the mouth. [NIH]

Lobe: A more or less well-defined portion of any organ, especially of the brain, lungs, and glands. Lobes are demarcated by fissures, sulci, connective tissue, and by their shape. [EU]

Malformation: A morphologic defect resulting from an intrinsically abnormal developmental process. [EU]

Mandible: The largest and strongest bone of the FACE constituting the lower jaw. It supports the lower teeth. [NIH]

Neonatal: Pertaining to the first four weeks after birth. [EU]

Neural: 1. Pertaining to a nerve or to the nerves. 2. Situated in the region of the spinal axis, as the neutral arch. [EU]

Neuroanatomy: Study of the anatomy of the nervous system as a specialty or discipline. [NIH]

Neurology: A medical specialty concerned with the study of the structures, functions, and diseases of the nervous system. [NIH]

Neuronal: Pertaining to a neuron or neurons (= conducting cells of the nervous system). [EU]

Neurons: The basic cellular units of nervous tissue. Each neuron consists of a body, an axon, and dendrites. Their purpose is to receive, conduct, and transmit impulses in the nervous system. [NIH]

Niacin: Water-soluble vitamin of the B complex occurring in various animal and plant tissues. Required by the body for the formation of coenzymes NAD and NADP. Has pellagra-curative, vasodilating, and antilipemic properties. [NIH]

Oral: Pertaining to the mouth, taken through or applied in the mouth, as an oral medication or an oral thermometer. [EU]

Overdose: 1. To administer an excessive dose. 2. An excessive dose. [EU]

Paralysis: Loss or impairment of motor function in a part due to lesion of the neural or muscular mechanism; also by analogy, impairment of sensory function (sensory paralysis). In addition to the types named below, paralysis is further distinguished as traumatic, syphilitic, toxic, etc., according to its cause; or as obturator, ulnar, etc., according to the nerve part, or muscle specially affected. [EU]

Parasitic: Pertaining to, of the nature of, or caused by a parasite. [EU]

Parietal: 1. Of or pertaining to the walls of a cavity. 2. Pertaining to or located near the parietal bone, as the parietal lobe. [EU]

Pediatrics: A medical specialty concerned with maintaining health and providing medical care to children from birth to adolescence. [NIH]

Posterior: Situated in back of, or in the back part of, or affecting the back or dorsal surface of the body. In lower animals, it refers to the caudal end of the body. [EU]

Potassium: An element that is in the alkali group of metals. It has an atomic symbol K, atomic number 19, and atomic weight 39.10. It is the chief cation in the intracellular fluid of muscle and other cells. Potassium ion is a strong electrolyte and it plays a significant role in the regulation of fluid volume and maintenance of the water-electrolyte balance. [NIH]

Progressive: Advancing; going forward; going from bad to worse; increasing in scope or severity. [EU]

Prosencephalon: The part of the brain developed from the most rostral of the three primary vesicles of the embryonic neural tube and consisting of the diencephalon and telencephalon. [NIH]

Proteins: Polymers of amino acids linked by peptide bonds. The specific sequence of amino acids determines the shape and function of the protein. [NIH]

Psychiatric: Pertaining to or within the purview of psychiatry. [EU]

Psychomotor: Pertaining to motor effects of cerebral or psychic activity. [EU]

Quadriplegia: Severe or complete loss of motor function in all four limbs which may result from brain diseases; spinal cord diseases; peripheral nervous system diseases; neuromuscular diseases; or rarely muscular diseases. The locked-in syndrome is characterized by quadriplegia in combination with cranial muscle paralysis. Consciousness is spared and the only retained voluntary motor activity may be limited eye movements. This condition is usually caused by a lesion in the upper brain stem which injures the descending cortico-spinal and cortico-bulbar tracts. [NIH]

Reflex: 1. Reflected. 2. A reflected action or movement; the sum total of any particular involuntary activity. [EU]

Riboflavin: Nutritional factor found in milk, eggs, malted barley, liver, kidney, heart, and leafy vegetables. The richest natural source is yeast. It occurs in the free form only in the retina of the eye, in whey, and in urine; its principal forms in tissues and cells are as FMN and FAD. [NIH]

Rubella: An acute, usually benign, infectious disease caused by a togavirus and most often affecting children and nonimmune young adults, in which the virus enters the respiratory tract via droplet nuclei and spreads to the lymphatic system. It is characterized by a slight cold, sore throat, and fever, followed by enlargement of the postauricular, suboccipital, and cervical lymph nodes, and the appearances of a fine pink rash that begins on the head and spreads to become generalized. Called also German measles, roetln, röteln, and three-day measles, and rubeola in French and Spanish. [EU]

Sclerosis: A induration, or hardening; especially hardening of a part from inflammation and in diseases of the interstitial substance. The term is used chiefly for such a hardening of the nervous system due to hyperplasia of the connective tissue or to designate hardening of the blood vessels. [EU]

Seizures: Clinical or subclinical disturbances of cortical function due to a sudden, abnormal, excessive, and disorganized discharge of brain cells. Clinical manifestations include abnormal motor, sensory and psychic phenomena. Recurrent seizures are usually referred to as EPILEPSY or "seizure disorder." [NIH]

Selenium: An element with the atomic symbol Se, atomic number 34, and atomic weight 78.96. It is an essential micronutrient for mammals and other animals but is toxic in large amounts. Selenium protects intracellular structures against oxidative damage. It is an essential component of glutathione peroxidase. [NIH]

Shunt: 1. To turn to one side; to divert; to bypass. 2. A passage or anastomosis between two natural channels, especially between blood vessels. Such structures may be formed physiologically (e.g. to bypass a thrombosis) or they may be structural anomalies. 3. a surgically created anastomosis; also, the operation of forming a shunt. [EU]

Skull: The skeleton of the head including the bones of the face and the bones enclosing the brain. [NIH]

Spastic: 1. Of the nature of or characterized by spasms. 2. Hypertonic, so that the muscles are stiff and the movements awkward. 3. A person exhibiting spasticity, such as occurs in spastic paralysis or in cerebral palsy. [EU]

Spectrum: A charted band of wavelengths of electromagnetic vibrations obtained by refraction and diffraction. By extension, a measurable range of activity, such as the range of bacteria affected by an antibiotic (antibacterial s.) or the complete range of manifestations of a disease. [EU]

Symptomatic: 1. Pertaining to or of the nature of a symptom. 2. Indicative (of a particular disease or disorder). 3. Exhibiting the symptoms of a particular disease but having a different cause. 4. Directed at the allying of symptoms, as symptomatic treatment. [EU]

Thermoregulation: Heat regulation. [EU]

Thyroxine: An amino acid of the thyroid gland which exerts a stimulating effect on thyroid metabolism. [NIH]

Tomography: The recording of internal body images at a predetermined plane by means of the tomograph; called also body section roentgenography. [EU]

Tone: 1. The normal degree of vigour and tension; in muscle, the resistance to passive elongation or stretch; tonus. 2. A particular quality of sound or of voice. 3. To make permanent, or to change, the colour of silver stain by chemical treatment, usually with a heavy metal. [EU]

Torticollis: Wryneck; a contracted state of the cervical muscles, producing twisting of the neck and an unnatural position of the head. [EU]

Toxic: Pertaining to, due to, or of the nature of a poison or toxin; manifesting the symptoms of severe infection. [EU]

Toxin: A poison; frequently used to refer specifically to a protein produced by some higher plants, certain animals, and pathogenic bacteria, which is highly toxic for other living organisms. Such substances are differentiated from the simple chemical poisons and the vegetable alkaloids by their high molecular weight and antigenicity. [EU]

Transillumination: Passage of light through body tissues or cavities for examination of internal structures. [NIH]

Trisomy: The possession of a third chromosome of any one type in an otherwise diploid cell. [NIH]

Ultrasonography: The visualization of deep structures of the body by recording the reflections of echoes of pulses of ultrasonic waves directed into the tissues. Use of ultrasound for imaging or diagnostic purposes employs frequencies ranging from 1.6 to 10 megahertz. [NIH]

Vascular: Pertaining to blood vessels or indicative of a copious blood supply. [EU]

Vasculitis: Inflammation of a vessel, angiitis. [EU]

Viral: Pertaining to, caused by, or of the nature of virus. [EU]

General Dictionaries and Glossaries

While the above glossary is essentially complete, the dictionaries listed here cover virtually all aspects of medicine, from basic words and phrases to more advanced terms (sorted alphabetically by title; hyperlinks provide rankings, information and reviews at Amazon.com):

- **Dictionary of Medical Acronymns & Abbreviations** by Stanley Jablonski (Editor), Paperback, 4th edition (2001), Lippincott Williams & Wilkins Publishers, ISBN: 1560534605, **http://www.amazon.com/exec/obidos/ASIN/1560534605/icongroupinterna**
- **Dictionary of Medical Terms : For the Nonmedical Person (Dictionary of Medical Terms for the Nonmedical Person, Ed 4)** by Mikel A. Rothenberg, M.D, et al, Paperback - 544 pages, 4th edition (2000), Barrons Educational Series, ISBN: 0764112015, **http://www.amazon.com/exec/obidos/ASIN/0764112015/icongroupinterna**
- **A Dictionary of the History of Medicine** by A. Sebastian, CD-Rom edition (2001), CRC Press-Parthenon Publishers, ISBN: 185070368X, **http://www.amazon.com/exec/obidos/ASIN/185070368X/icongroupinterna**
- **Dorland's Illustrated Medical Dictionary (Standard Version)** by Dorland, et al, Hardcover - 2088 pages, 29th edition (2000), W B Saunders Co, ISBN: 0721662544, **http://www.amazon.com/exec/obidos/ASIN/0721662544/icongroupinterna**
- **Dorland's Electronic Medical Dictionary** by Dorland, et al, Software, 29th Book & CD-Rom edition (2000), Harcourt Health Sciences, ISBN: 0721694934,

http://www.amazon.com/exec/obidos/ASIN/0721694934/icongroupinterna

- **Dorland's Pocket Medical Dictionary (Dorland's Pocket Medical Dictionary, 26th Ed)** Hardcover - 912 pages, 26th edition (2001), W B Saunders Co, ISBN: 0721682812, **http://www.amazon.com/exec/obidos/ASIN/0721682812/icongroupinterna/103-4193558-7304618**
- **Melloni's Illustrated Medical Dictionary (Melloni's Illustrated Medical Dictionary, 4th Ed)** by Melloni, Hardcover, 4th edition (2001), CRC Press-Parthenon Publishers, ISBN: 85070094X, **http://www.amazon.com/exec/obidos/ASIN/85070094X/icongroupinterna**
- **Stedman's Electronic Medical Dictionary Version 5.0 (CD-ROM for Windows and Macintosh, Individual)** by Stedmans, CD-ROM edition (2000), Lippincott Williams & Wilkins Publishers, ISBN: 0781726328, **http://www.amazon.com/exec/obidos/ASIN/0781726328/icongroupinterna**
- **Stedman's Medical Dictionary** by Thomas Lathrop Stedman, Hardcover - 2098 pages, 27th edition (2000), Lippincott, Williams & Wilkins, ISBN: 068340007X, **http://www.amazon.com/exec/obidos/ASIN/068340007X/icongroupinterna**
- **Tabers Cyclopedic Medical Dictionary (Thumb Index)** by Donald Venes (Editor), et al, Hardcover - 2439 pages, 19th edition (2001), F A Davis Co, ISBN: 0803606540, **http://www.amazon.com/exec/obidos/ASIN/0803606540/icongroupinterna**

INDEX

Lightning Source UK Ltd.
Milton Keynes UK
UKOW020616270113

205403UK00003B/204/A